KU-301-552

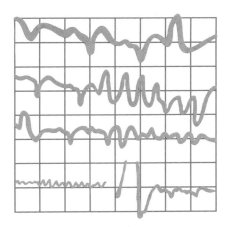

The
ECG
Made Easy

For *Elsevier*
Content Strategist: Laurence Hunter
Content Development Specialist: Helen Leng
Project Manager: Louisa Talbott and Helius
Designer/Design Direction: Helius and Mark Rogers
Illustration Manager: Jennifer Rose
Illustrators: Helius and Gecko Ltd

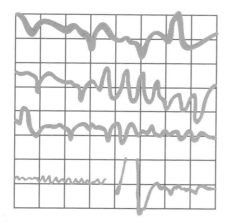

The
ECG
Made Easy

EIGHTH EDITION

John R. Hampton
DM MA DPhil FRCP FFPM FESC

Emeritus Professor of Cardiology
University of Nottingham, UK

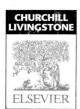

EDINBURGH LONDON NEW YORK OXFORD PHILADELPHIA ST LOUIS SYDNEY TORONTO 2013

CHURCHILL LIVINGSTONE
ELSEVIER

© 2013 Elsevier Ltd. All rights reserved.

No part of this publication may be reproduced or transmitted in any form or by any means, electronic or mechanical, including photocopying, recording, or any information storage and retrieval system, without permission in writing from the publisher. Details on how to seek permission, further information about the publisher's permissions policies and our arrangements with organizations such as the Copyright Clearance Center and the Copyright Licensing Agency, can be found at our website: www.elsevier.com/permissions.

This book and the individual contributions contained in it are protected under copyright by the publisher (other than as may be noted herein).

First edition 1973
Second edition 1980
Third edition 1986
Fourth edition 1992
Fifth edition 1997
Sixth edition 2003
Seventh edition 2008
Eighth edition 2013

ISBN 978-0-7020-4641-4
  Reprinted 2014
International ISBN 978-0-7020-4642-1
  Reprinted 2013, 2014
e-book ISBN 978-0-7020-5243-9

British Library Cataloguing in Publication Data
A catalogue record for this book is available from the British Library

Library of Congress Cataloging in Publication Data
A catalog record for this book is available from the Library of Congress

Notices

Knowledge and best practice in this field are constantly changing. As new research and experience broaden our understanding, changes in research methods, professional practices, or medical treatment may become necessary.

Practitioners and researchers must always rely on their own experience and knowledge in evaluating and using any information, methods, compounds, or experiments described herein. In using such information or methods they should be mindful of their own safety and the safety of others, including parties for whom they have a professional responsibility.

With respect to any drug or pharmaceutical products identified, readers are advised to check the most current information provided (i) on procedures featured or (ii) by the manufacturer of each product to be administered, to verify the recommended dose or formula, the method and duration of administration, and contraindications. It is the responsibility of practitioners, relying on their own experience and knowledge of their patients, to make diagnoses, to determine dosages and the best treatment for each individual patient, and to take all appropriate safety precautions.

To the fullest extent of the law, neither the publisher nor the author assumes any liability for any injury and/or damage to persons or property as a matter of products liability, negligence or otherwise, or from any use or operation of any methods, products, instructions, or ideas contained in the material herein.

ELSEVIER your source for books, journals and multimedia in the health sciences

www.elsevierhealth.com

  Working together to grow libraries in developing countries

www.elsevier.com • www.bookaid.org

The Publisher's policy is to use paper manufactured from sustainable forests

Printed in China

Preface

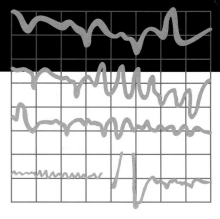

The ECG Made Easy was first published in 1973, and well over half a million copies of the first seven editions have been sold. The book has been translated into German, French, Spanish, Italian, Portuguese, Polish, Czech, Indonesian, Japanese, Russian and Turkish, and into two Chinese languages. The aims of this edition are the same as before: the book is not intended to be a comprehensive textbook of electrophysiology, nor even of ECG interpretation – it is designed as an introduction to the ECG for medical students, technicians, nurses and paramedics. It may also provide useful revision for those who have forgotten what they learned as students.

There really is no need for the ECG to be daunting: just as most people drive a car without knowing much about engines, and gardeners do not need to be botanists, most people can make full use of the ECG without becoming submerged in its complexities. This book encourages the reader to accept that the ECG is easy to understand and that its use is just a natural extension of taking the patient's history and performing a physical examination.

The first edition of The ECG Made Easy (1973) was described by the British Medical Journal as a 'medical classic'. The book has been a favourite of generations of medical students and nurses, and it has changed a lot through progressive editions. This eighth edition differs from its predecessors in that it has been divided into two parts. The first part, 'The Basics' explains the ECG in the simplest possible terms, and can be read on its own. It focuses on the fundamentals of ECG recording, reporting and interpretation, including the classical ECG abnormalities. The second part, 'Making the most of the ECG', has been expanded and divided into three chapters. It makes the point that an ECG is simply a tool for the diagnosis and treatment of patients, and so has to be interpreted in the light of the history and physical examination of the patient from whom it was recorded. The variations that might be encountered in the situations in which the ECG is most commonly used are considered in separate chapters on healthy subjects (where there is a wide range of normality) and on patients presenting with chest pain, breathlessness, palpitations or syncope. The book is longer than the previous editions, but that does not mean that the ECG has become more difficult to understand.

The ECG Made Easy should help students to prepare for examinations, but for the development of clinical competence – and confidence – there is no substitute for reporting on large numbers of clinical records. Two companion texts may help those who have mastered *The ECG Made Easy* and want to progress further. *The ECG in Practice* deals with the relationship between the patient's history and physical signs and the ECG, and also with the many variations in the ECG seen in health and disease. *150 ECG Problems* describes 150 clinical cases and gives their full ECGs, in a format that encourages the reader to interpret the records and decide on treatment before looking at the answers.

I am extremely grateful to Mrs Alison Gale who has not only been a superb copy editor but who has also become an expert in ECG interpretation and has made a major contribution to this edition and to previous ones. The expertise of Helius has been crucial for the new layout of this 8th edition. I am also grateful to Laurence Hunter, Helen Leng and Louisa Talbott of Elsevier for their continuing support.

The title of *The ECG Made Easy* was suggested more than 30 years ago by the late Tony Mitchell, Foundation Professor of Medicine at the University of Nottingham, and many more books have been published with a 'Made Easy' title since then. I am grateful to him and to the many people who have helped to refine the book over the years, and particularly to many students for their constructive criticisms and helpful comments, which have reinforced my belief that the ECG really is easy to understand.

John Hampton
Nottingham, 2013

Contents

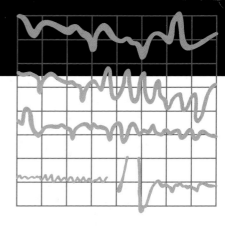

Further reading

The symbol

indicates cross-references to useful information in the book *The ECG in Practice*, 6th edn.

The basics

The fundamentals of ECG recording, reporting and interpretation

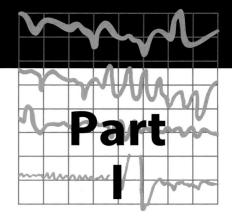

Part I

Before you can use the ECG as an aid to diagnosis or treatment, you have to understand the basics. Part I of this book explains why the electrical activity of the heart can be recorded as an ECG, and describes the significance of the 12 ECG 'leads' that make 'pictures' of the electrical activity seen from different directions.

Part I also explains how the ECG can be used to measure the heart rate, to assess the speed of electrical conduction through different parts of the heart, and to determine the rhythm of the heart. The causes of common 'abnormal' ECG patterns are described.

What the ECG is about

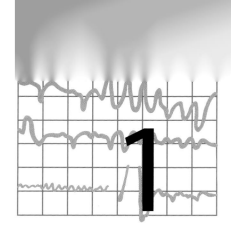

'ECG' stands for electrocardiogram, or electrocardiograph. In some countries, the abbreviation used is 'EKG'. Remember:

- By the time you have finished this book, you should be able to say and mean 'The ECG is easy to understand'.
- Most abnormalities of the ECG are amenable to reason.

WHAT TO EXPECT FROM THE ECG

Clinical diagnosis depends mainly on a patient's history, and to a lesser extent on the physical examination. The ECG can provide evidence to support a diagnosis, and in some cases it is crucial for patient management. It is, however, important to see the ECG as a tool, and not as an end in itself.

The ECG is essential for the diagnosis, and therefore the management, of abnormal cardiac rhythms. It helps with the diagnosis of the cause of chest pain, and the proper use of early intervention in myocardial infarction depends upon it. It can help with the diagnosis of the cause of dizziness, syncope and breathlessness.

With practice, interpreting the ECG is a matter of pattern recognition. However, the ECG can be analysed from first principles if a few simple rules and basic facts are remembered. This chapter is about these rules and facts.

THE ELECTRICITY OF THE HEART

The contraction of any muscle is associated with electrical changes called 'depolarization', and these changes can be detected by electrodes attached to the surface of the body. Since all muscular contraction will be detected, the electrical changes associated with contraction of the heart muscle will only be clear if the patient is fully relaxed and no skeletal muscles are contracting.

Although the heart has four chambers, from the electrical point of view it can be thought of as having only two, because the two atria contract together ('depolarization'), and then the two ventricles contract together.

THE WIRING DIAGRAM OF THE HEART

The electrical discharge for each cardiac cycle normally starts in a special area of the right atrium called the 'sinoatrial (SA) node' (Fig. 1.1). Depolarization then spreads through the atrial muscle fibres. There is a delay while depolarization spreads through another special area in the atrium, the 'atrioventricular node' (also called the 'AV node', or sometimes just 'the node'). Thereafter, the depolarization wave travels very rapidly down specialized conduction tissue, the 'bundle of His', which divides in the septum between the ventricles into right and left bundle branches. The left bundle branch itself divides into two. Within the mass of ventricular muscle, conduction spreads somewhat more slowly, through specialized tissue called 'Purkinje fibres'.

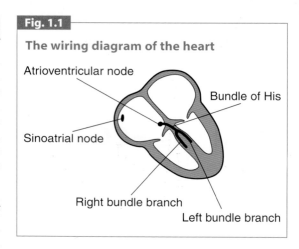

Fig. 1.1

The wiring diagram of the heart

Atrioventricular node

Bundle of His

Sinoatrial node

Right bundle branch

Left bundle branch

THE RHYTHM OF THE HEART

As we shall see later, electrical activation of the heart can sometimes begin in places other than the SA node. The word 'rhythm' is used to refer to the part of the heart which is controlling the activation sequence. The normal heart rhythm, with electrical activation beginning in the SA node, is called 'sinus rhythm'.

THE DIFFERENT PARTS OF THE ECG

The muscle mass of the atria is small compared with that of the ventricles, and so the electrical change accompanying the contraction of the atria is small. Contraction of the atria is associated with the ECG wave called 'P' (Fig. 1.2). The

Fig. 1.2

Shape of the normal ECG, including a U wave

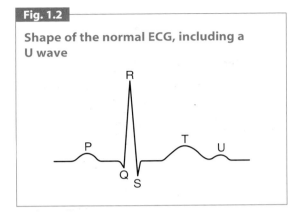

The letters P, Q, R, S and T were selected in the early days of ECG history, and were chosen arbitrarily. The P Q, R, S and T deflections are all called waves; the Q, R and S waves together make up a complex; and the interval between the S wave and the beginning of the T wave is called the ST 'segment'.

In some ECGs an extra wave can be seen on the end of the T wave, and this is called a U wave. Its origin is uncertain, though it may represent repolarization of the papillary muscles. If a U wave follows a normally shaped T wave, it can be assumed to be normal. If it follows a flattened T wave, it may be pathological (see Ch. 4).

The different parts of the QRS complex are labelled as shown in Figure 1.3. If the first deflection is downward, it is called a Q wave (Fig. 1.3a). An upward deflection is called an R wave, regardless of whether it is preceded by a Q wave or not (Figs 1.3b and 1.3c). Any deflection below the baseline following an R wave is called an S wave, regardless of whether there is a preceding Q wave (Figs 1.3d and 1.3e).

ventricular mass is large, and so there is a large deflection of the ECG when the ventricles are depolarized: this is called the 'QRS' complex. The 'T' wave of the ECG is associated with the return of the ventricular mass to its resting electrical state ('repolarization').

Fig. 1.3

Parts of the QRS complex

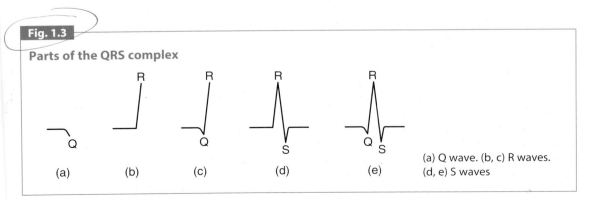

(a) Q wave. (b, c) R waves. (d, e) S waves

TIMES AND SPEEDS

ECG machines record changes in electrical activity by drawing a trace on a moving paper strip. ECG machines run at a standard rate of 25 mm/s and use paper with standard-sized squares. Each large square (5 mm) represents 0.2 second (s), i.e. 200 milliseconds (ms) (Fig. 1.4). Therefore, there are five large squares per second, and 300 per minute. So an ECG event, such as a QRS complex, occurring once per large square is occurring at a rate of 300/min. The heart rate can be calculated rapidly by remembering the sequence in Table 1.1.

Just as the length of paper between R waves gives the heart rate, so the distance between the different parts of the P–QRS–T complex shows the time taken for conduction of the electrical discharge to spread through the different parts of the heart.

The PR interval is measured from the beginning of the P wave to the beginning of the QRS complex, and it is the time taken for excitation to spread from the SA node, through the atrial muscle and the AV node, down the bundle of His and into the ventricular muscle. Logically, it should be called the PQ interval, but common usage is 'PR interval' (Fig. 1.5).

The normal PR interval is 120–220 ms, represented by 3–5 small squares. Most of this time is taken up by delay in the AV node (Fig. 1.6).

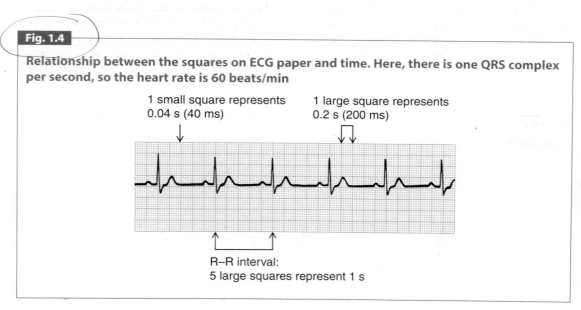

Fig. 1.4

Relationship between the squares on ECG paper and time. Here, there is one QRS complex per second, so the heart rate is 60 beats/min

1 small square represents 0.04 s (40 ms)

1 large square represents 0.2 s (200 ms)

R–R interval:
5 large squares represent 1 s

Fig. 1.5

The components of the ECG complex

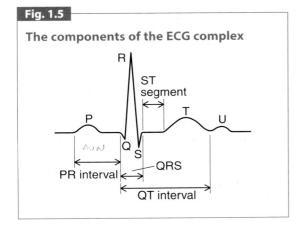

Table 1.1 **Relationship between the number of large squares between successive R waves and the heart rate**

R–R interval (large squares)	Heart rate (beats/min)
1	300
2	150
3	100
4	75
5	60
6	50

If the PR interval is very short, either the atria have been depolarized from close to the AV node, or there is abnormally fast conduction from the atria to the ventricles.

The duration of the QRS complex shows how long excitation takes to spread through the ventricles. The QRS complex duration is normally 120 ms (represented by three small

Fig. 1.6

Normal PR interval and QRS complex

PR
0.18 s (180 ms)

QRS
0.12 s (120 ms)

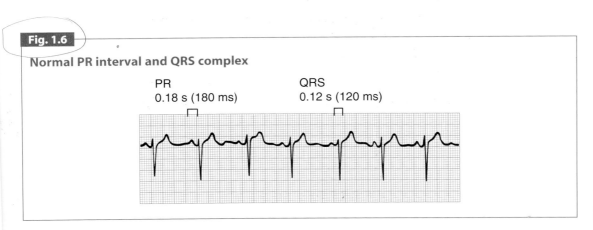

7

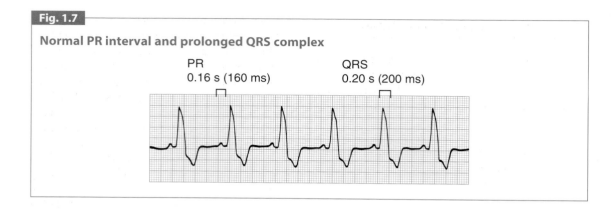

Fig. 1.7

Normal PR interval and prolonged QRS complex

PR
0.16 s (160 ms)

QRS
0.20 s (200 ms)

squares) or less, but any abnormality of conduction takes longer, and causes widened QRS complexes (Fig. 1.7). Remember that the QRS complex represents depolarization, not contraction, of the ventricles – contraction is proceeding during the ECG's ST segment.

The QT interval varies with the heart rate. It is prolonged in patients with some electrolyte abnormalities, and more importantly it is prolonged by some drugs. A prolonged QT interval (greater than 450 ms) may lead to ventricular tachycardia.

CALIBRATION

A limited amount of information is given by the height of the P waves, QRS complexes and T waves, provided the machine is properly

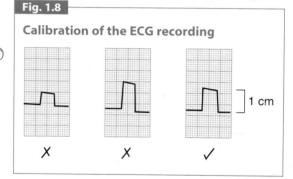

Fig. 1.8

Calibration of the ECG recording

1 cm

✗   ✗   ✓

calibrated. A standard signal of 1 millivolt (mV) should move the stylus vertically 1 cm (two large squares) (Fig. 1.8), and this 'calibration' signal should be included with every record.

THE ECG – ELECTRICAL PICTURES

The word 'lead' sometimes causes confusion. Sometimes it is used to mean the pieces of wire that connect the patient to the ECG recorder. Properly, a lead is an electrical picture of the heart.

The electrical signal from the heart is detected at the surface of the body through electrodes, which are joined to the ECG recorder by wires. One electrode is attached to each limb, and six to the front of the chest.

The ECG recorder compares the electrical activity detected in the different electrodes, and the electrical picture so obtained is called a 'lead'. The different comparisons 'look at' the heart from different directions. For example, when the recorder is set to 'lead I' it is comparing the electrical events detected by the electrodes attached to the right and left arms. Each lead gives a different view of the electrical activity of the heart, and so a different ECG pattern. Strictly, each ECG pattern should be called 'lead ...', but often the word 'lead' is omitted.

The ECG is made up of 12 characteristic views of the heart, six obtained from the 'limb' leads (I, II, III, VR, VL, VF) and six from the 'chest' leads (V_1–V_6). It is not necessary to remember how the leads (or views of the heart) are derived by the recorder, but for those who like to know how it works, see Table 1.2. The electrode attached to the right leg is used as an earth, and does not contribute to any lead.

Table 1.2 ECG leads

Lead	Comparison of electrical activity
I	LA and RA
II	LL and RA
III	LL and LA
VR	RA and average of (LA + LL)
VL	LA and average of (RA + LL)
VF	LL and average of (LA + RA)
V_1	V_1 and average of (LA + RA + LL)
V_2	V_2 and average of (LA + RA + LL)
V_3	V_3 and average of (LA + RA + LL)
V_4	V_4 and average of (LA + RA + LL)
V_5	V_5 and average of (LA + RA + LL)
V_6	V_6 and average of (LA + RA + LL)

Key: LA, left arm; RA, right arm; LL, left leg.

THE 12-LEAD ECG

ECG interpretation is easy if you remember the directions from which the various leads look at the heart. The six 'standard' leads, which are recorded from the electrodes attached to the limbs, can be thought of as looking at the heart in a vertical plane (i.e. from the sides or the feet) (Fig. 1.9).

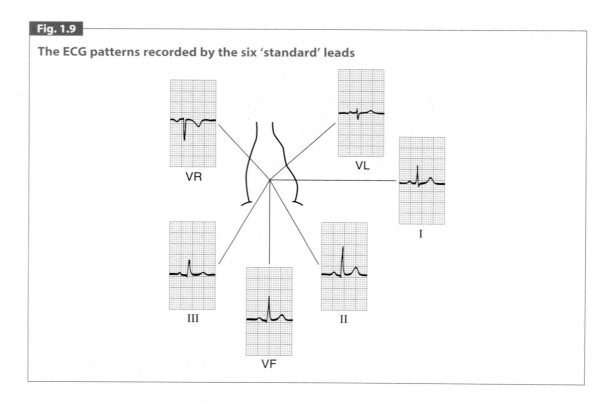

Fig. 1.9

The ECG patterns recorded by the six 'standard' leads

Leads I, II and VL look at the left lateral surface of the heart, leads III and VF at the inferior surface, and lead VR looks at the right atrium.

The six V leads (V₁–V₆) look at the heart in a horizontal plane, from the front and the left side. Thus, leads V_1 and V_2 look at the right ventricle, V_3 and V_4 look at the septum between the ventricles and the anterior wall of the left ventricle, and V_5 and V_6 look at the anterior and lateral walls of the left ventricle (Fig. 1.10).

Fig. 1.10

The relationship between the six chest leads and the heart

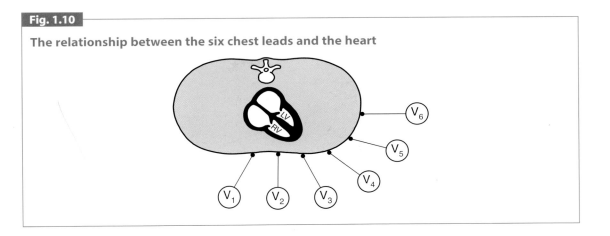

As with the limb leads, the chest leads each show a different ECG pattern (Fig. 1.11). In each lead the pattern is characteristic, being similar in individuals who have normal hearts.

The cardiac rhythm is identified from whichever lead shows the P wave most clearly – usually lead II. When a single lead is recorded simply to show the rhythm, it is called a 'rhythm strip', but it is important not to make any diagnosis from a single lead, other than identifying the cardiac rhythm.

THE SHAPE OF THE QRS COMPLEX

We now need to consider why the ECG has a characteristic appearance in each lead.

THE QRS COMPLEX IN THE LIMB LEADS

The ECG machine is arranged so that when a depolarization wave spreads towards a lead the stylus moves upwards, and when it spreads away from the lead the stylus moves downwards.

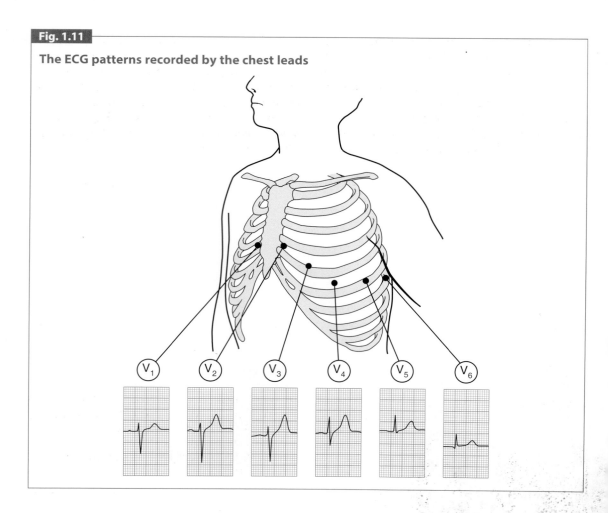

Fig. 1.11

The ECG patterns recorded by the chest leads

Depolarization spreads through the heart in many directions at once, but the shape of the QRS complex shows the average direction in which the wave of depolarization is spreading through the ventricles (Fig. 1.12).

If the QRS complex is predominantly upward, or positive (i.e. the R wave is greater than the S wave), the depolarization is moving towards that lead (Fig. 1.12a). If predominantly downward, or negative (the S wave is greater than the R wave), the depolarization is moving away from that lead (Fig. 1.12b). When the depolarization wave is moving at right angles to the lead, the R and S waves are of equal size (Fig. 1.12c). Q waves, when present, have a special significance, which we shall discuss later.

Fig. 1.12

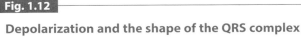

Depolarization and the shape of the QRS complex

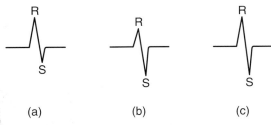

Depolarization (a) moving towards the lead, causing a predominantly upward QRS complex; (b) moving away from the lead, causing a predominantly downward QRS complex; and (c) at right angles to the lead, generating equal R and S waves

THE CARDIAC AXIS

Leads VR and II look at the heart from opposite directions. When seen from the front, the depolarization wave normally spreads through the ventricles from 11 o'clock to 5 o'clock, so the deflections in lead VR are normally mainly downward (negative) and in lead II mainly upward (positive) (Fig. 1.13).

The average direction of spread of the depolarization wave through the ventricles as seen from the front is called the 'cardiac axis'. It is useful to decide whether this axis is in a normal direction or not. The direction of the axis can be derived most easily from the QRS complex in leads I, II and III.

A normal 11 o'clock–5 o'clock axis means that the depolarizing wave is spreading towards leads I, II and III, and is therefore associated with a predominantly upward deflection in all these leads; the deflection will be greater in lead II than in I or III (Fig. 1.14).

When the R and S waves of the QRS complex are equal, the cardiac axis is at right angles to that lead.

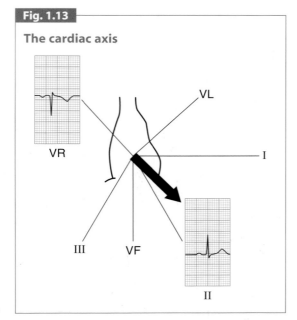

Fig. 1.13

The cardiac axis

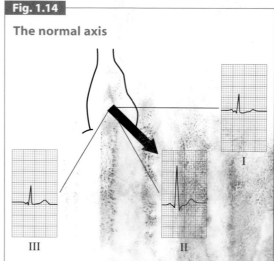

Fig. 1.14

The normal axis

If the right ventricle becomes hypertrophied, it has more effect on the QRS complex than the left ventricle, and the average depolarization wave – the axis – will swing towards the right. The deflection in lead I becomes negative (predominantly downward) because depolarization is spreading away from it, and the deflection in lead III becomes more positive (predominantly upward) because depolarization is spreading towards it (Fig. 1.15). This is called 'right axis deviation'. It is associated mainly with pulmonary conditions that put a strain on the right side of the heart, and with congenital heart disorders.

When the left ventricle becomes hypertrophied, it exerts more influence on the QRS complex than the right ventricle. Hence, the axis may swing to the left, and the QRS complex becomes predominantly negative in lead III (Fig. 1.16). 'Left axis deviation' is not significant until the QRS complex deflection is also predominantly negative in lead II. Although left axis deviation can be due to excess influence of an enlarged left ventricle, in fact this axis change is usually due to a conduction defect rather than to increased bulk of the left ventricular muscle (see Ch. 2).

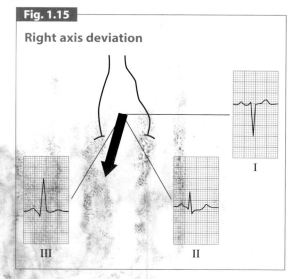

Fig. 1.15

Right axis deviation

III   II   I

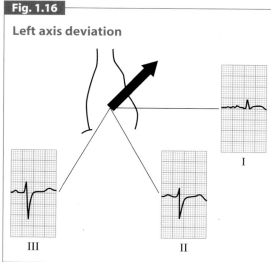

Fig. 1.16

Left axis deviation

III   II   I

The cardiac axis is sometimes measured in degrees (Fig. 1.17), though this is not clinically particularly useful. Lead I is taken as looking at the heart from 0°; lead II from +60°; lead VF from +90°; and lead III from +120°. Leads VL and VR look from −30° and −150°, respectively.

The normal cardiac axis is in the range −30° to +90°. If in lead II the S wave is greater than the R wave, the axis must be more than 90° away from lead II. In other words, it must be at a greater angle than −30°, and closer to the vertical (see Figs 1.16 and 1.17), and left axis deviation is present. Similarly, if the size of the R wave equals that of the S wave in lead I, the axis is at right angles to lead I or at +90°. This is the limit of normality towards the 'right'. If the S wave is greater than the R wave in lead I, the axis is at an angle of greater than +90°, and right axis deviation is present (Fig. 1.15).

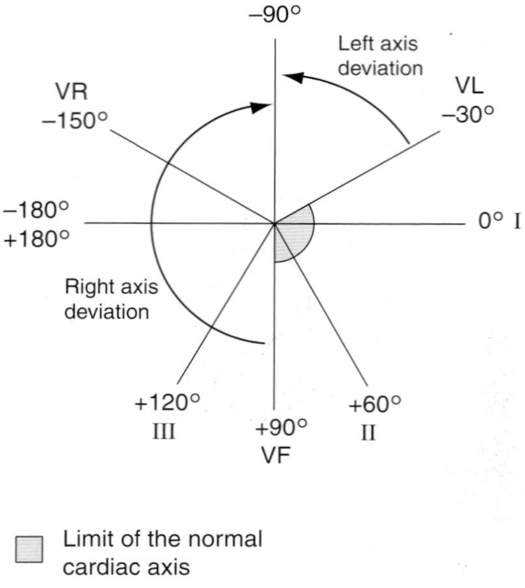

WHY WORRY ABOUT THE CARDIAC AXIS?

Right and left axis deviation in themselves are seldom significant – minor degrees occur in tall, thin individuals and in short, fat individuals, respectively. However, the presence of axis deviation should alert you to look for other signs of right and left ventricular hypertrophy (see Ch. 4). A change in axis to the right may suggest a pulmonary embolus, and a change to the left indicates a conduction defect.

THE QRS COMPLEX IN THE V LEADS

The shape of the QRS complex in the chest (V) leads is determined by two things:

- The septum between the ventricles is depolarized before the walls of the ventricles, and the depolarization wave spreads across the septum from left to right.
- In the normal heart there is more muscle in the wall of the left ventricle than in that of the right ventricle, and so the left ventricle exerts more influence on the ECG pattern than does the right ventricle.

Fig. 1.17

The cardiac axis and lead angles

−90°

Left axis deviation

VR −150°

VL −30°

−180° +180°

0° I

Right axis deviation

+120° III

+90° VF

+60° II

Limit of the normal cardiac axis

Leads V_1 and V_2 look at the right ventricle; leads V_3 and V_4 look at the septum; and leads V_5 and V_6 at the left ventricle (Fig. 1.10).

In a right ventricular lead the deflection is first upwards (R wave) as the septum is depolarized. In a left ventricular lead the opposite pattern is seen: there is a small downward deflection ('septal' Q wave) (Fig. 1.18).

In a right ventricular lead there is then a downward deflection (S wave) as the main muscle mass is depolarized – the electrical effects in the bigger left ventricle (in which depolarization is spreading away from a right ventricular lead) outweighing those in the smaller right ventricle.

In a left ventricular lead there is an upward deflection (R wave) as the ventricular muscle is depolarized (Fig. 1.19).

When the whole of the myocardium is depolarized, the ECG trace returns to the baseline (Fig. 1.20).

The QRS complex in the chest leads shows a progression from lead V_1, where it is predominantly downward, to lead V_6, where it is predominantly upward (Fig. 1.21). The 'transition point', where the R and S waves are equal, indicates the position of the interventricular septum.

Fig. 1.18

Shape of the QRS complex: first stage

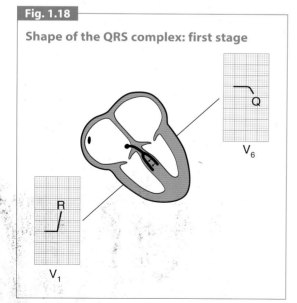

Fig. 1.19

Shape of the QRS complex: second stage

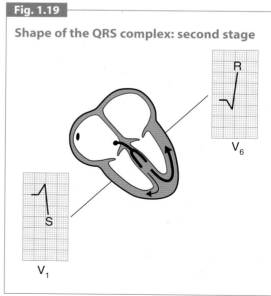

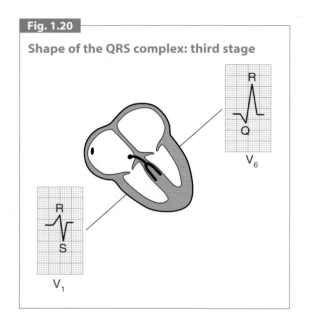

Fig. 1.20

Shape of the QRS complex: third stage

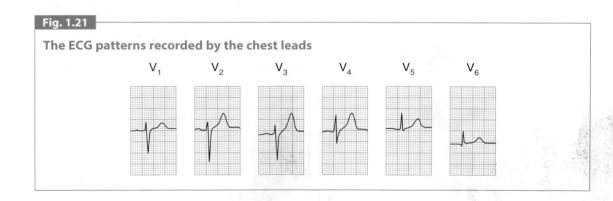

Fig. 1.21

The ECG patterns recorded by the chest leads

V_1 V_2 V_3 V_4 V_5 V_6

WHY WORRY ABOUT THE TRANSITION POINT?

If the right ventricle is enlarged, and occupies more of the precordium than is normal, the transition point will move from its normal position of leads V_3/V_4 to leads V_4/V_5 or sometimes leads V_5/V_6. Seen from below, the heart can be thought of as having rotated in a clockwise direction. 'Clockwise rotation' in the ECG is characteristic of chronic lung disease.

MAKING A RECORDING – PRACTICAL POINTS

Now that you know what an ECG should look like, and why it looks the way it does, we need to think about the practical side of making a recording. Some, but not all, ECG recorders produce a 'rhythm strip', which is a continuous record, usually of lead II. This is particularly useful when the rhythm is not normal. The next series of ECGs were all recorded from a healthy subject whose 'ideal' ECG is shown in Figure 1.22.

It is really important to make sure that the electrode marked LA is indeed attached to the left arm, RA to the right arm and so on. If the limb electrodes are wrongly attached, the 12-lead ECG will look very odd (Fig. 1.23). It is possible to interpret the ECG, but it is easier to recognize that there has been a mistake, and to repeat the recording.

Reversal of the leg electrodes does not make much difference to the ECG.

The chest electrodes need to be accurately positioned, so that abnormal patterns in the V leads can be identified, and so that records taken on different occasions can be compared. Identify the second rib interspace by feeling for the sternal angle – this is the point where the manubrium and the body of the sternum meet, and there is usually a palpable ridge where the body of the sternum begins, angling downwards in comparison to the manubrium. The second rib is attached to the sternum at the angle, and the second rib space is just below this. Having identified the second space, feel downwards for the third and then the fourth rib spaces, over which the electrodes for V_1 and V_2 are attached, to the right and left of the sternum, respectively.

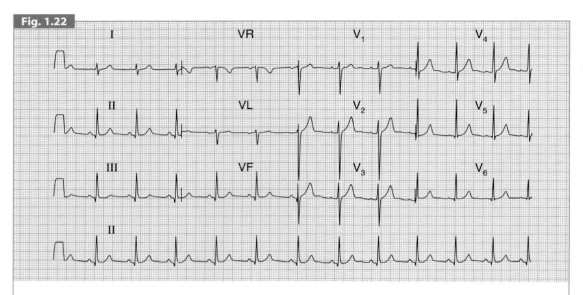

Fig. 1.22

A good record of a normal ECG
Note
- The upper three traces show the six limb leads (I, II, III, VR, VL, VF) and then the six chest leads
- The bottom trace is a 'rhythm strip', entirely recorded from lead II (i.e. no lead changes)
- The trace is clear, with P waves, QRS complexes and T waves visible in all leads

Fig. 1.23

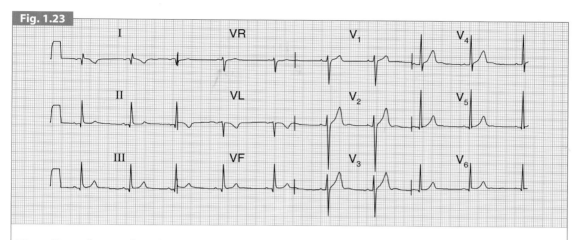

The effect of reversing the electrodes attached to the left and right arms
Note
- Compare with Figure 1.22, correctly recorded from the same patient
- Inverted P waves in lead I
- Abnormal QRS complexes and T waves in lead I
- Upright T waves in lead VR are most unusual

The other electrodes are then placed as shown in Figure 1.24, with V_4 in the midclavicular line (the imaginary vertical line starting from the midpoint of the clavicle); V_5 in the anterior axillary line (the line starting from the fold of skin that marks the front of the armpit); and V_6 in the midaxillary line.

Good electrical contact between the electrodes and the skin is essential. The effects on the ECG of poor skin contact are shown in Figure 1.25. The skin must be clean and dry – in any patient using creams or moisturizers (such as patients with skin disorders) it should be cleaned with alcohol; the alcohol must be

Fig. 1.24

The positions of the chest leads: note the fourth and fifth rib spaces

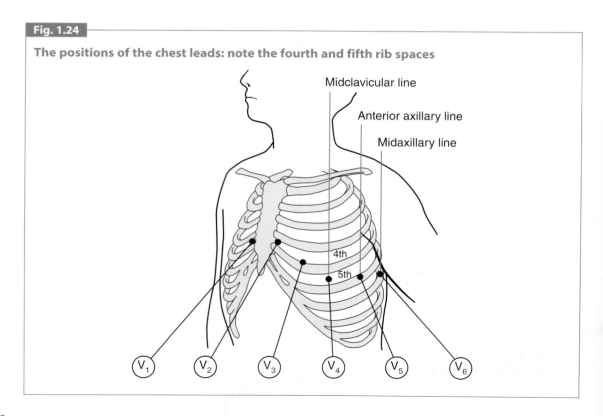

wiped off before the electrodes are applied. Abrasion of the skin is essential; in most patients all that is needed is a rub with a paper towel. In exercise testing, when the patient is likely to become sweaty, abrasive pads may be used – for these tests it is worth spending time to ensure good contact, because in many cases the ECG becomes almost unreadable towards the end of the test. Hair is a poor conductor of the electrical signal and prevents the electrodes from sticking to the skin. Shaving may be preferable, but patients may not like this – if the hair can be parted and firm contact made with the electrodes, this is acceptable. After

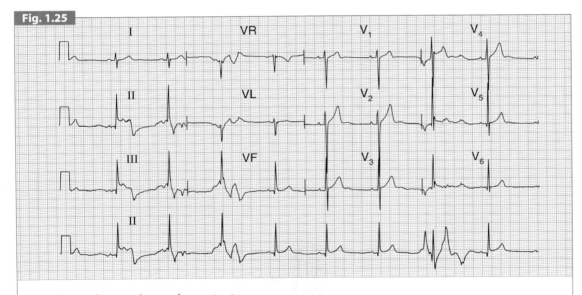

Fig. 1.25

The effect of poor electrode contact

Note

- Bizarre ECG patterns
- In the rhythm strip (lead II), the patterns vary

shaving, the skin will need to be cleaned with alcohol or a soapy wipe.

Even with the best of ECG recorders, electrical interference can cause regular oscillation in the ECG trace, at first sight giving the impression of a thickened baseline (Fig. 1.26). It can be extremely difficult to work out where electrical interference may be coming from, but think about electric lights, and electric motors on beds and mattresses.

ECG recorders are normally calibrated so that 1 mV of signal causes a deflection of 1 cm

Fig. 1.26

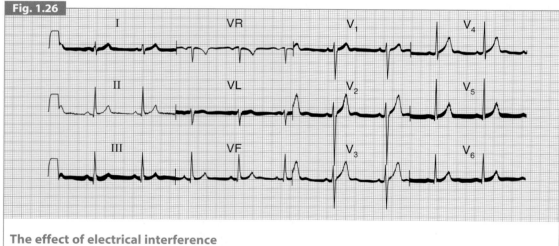

The effect of electrical interference

Note

• Regular sharp high-frequency spikes, giving the appearance of a thick baseline on the ECG paper, and a calibration signal usually appears at the beginning (and often also at the end) of a record. If the calibration setting is wrong, the ECG complexes will look too large or too small (Figs 1.27 and 1.28). Large complexes may be confused with left ventricular hypertrophy (see Ch. 4), and small complexes might suggest that there is something like a pericardial effusion reducing the electrical signal from the heart. So, check the calibration.

ECG recorders are normally set to run at a paper speed of 25 mm/s, but they can be altered

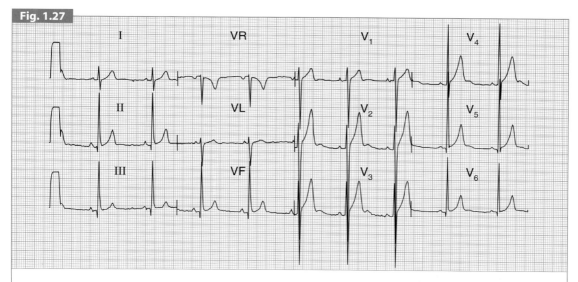

Fig. 1.27

The effect of over-calibration
Note
- The calibration signal (1 mV) at the left-hand end of each line causes a deflection of 2 cm
- All the complexes are large compared with an ECG recorded with the correct calibration (e.g. Fig. 1.22, in which 1 mV causes a deflection of 1 cm)

Fig. 1.28

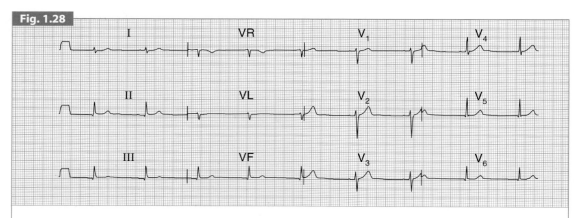

I   VR   V₁   V₄

II   VL   V₂   V₅

III   VF   V₃   V₆

The effect of under-calibration
Note
- The calibration signal (1 mV) causes a deflection of 0.5 cm
- All the complexes are small

to run at slower speeds (which make the complexes appear spiky and bunched together) or to 50 mm/s (Figs 1.29 and 1.30). The faster speed is used regularly in some European countries, and makes the ECG look 'spread out'. In theory this can make the P wave easier to see, but in fact flattening out the P wave tends to hide it, and so this fast speed is seldom useful.

ECG recorders are 'tuned' to the electrical frequency generated by heart muscle, but they will also detect the contraction of skeletal muscle. It is therefore essential that a patient is relaxed, warm and lying comfortably – if they are moving or shivering, or have involuntary movements such as those of Parkinson's disease, the recorder will pick up a lot of muscular activity, which in extreme cases can mask the ECG (Figs 1.31 and 1.32).

So, the ECG recorder will do most of the work for you – but remember to:

- attach the electrodes to the correct limbs
- ensure good electrical contact
- check the calibration and speed settings
- get the patient comfortable and relaxed.

Then just press the button, and the recorder will automatically provide a beautiful 12-lead ECG.

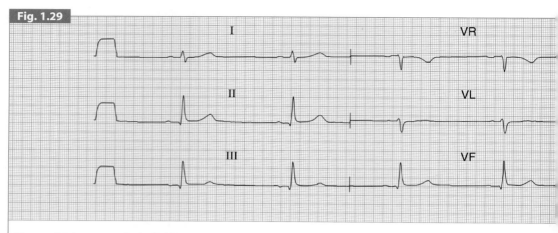

Fig. 1.29

Normal ECG recorded with a paper speed of 50 mm/s
Note
- A paper speed of 50 mm/s is faster than normal
- Long interval between QRS complexes gives the impression of a slow heart rate
- Widened QRS complexes
- Apparently very long QT interval

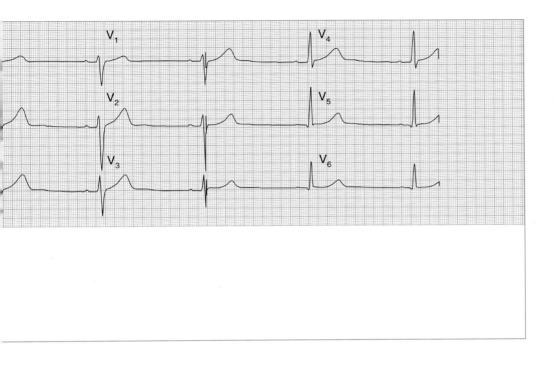

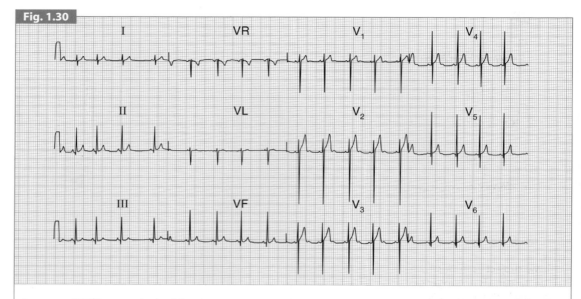

Fig. 1.30

A normal ECG recorded with a paper speed of 12.5 mm/s

Note
- A paper speed of 12.5 mm/s is slower than normal
- QRS complexes are close together, giving the impression of a rapid heart rate
- P waves, QRS complexes and T waves are all narrow and 'spiky'

Fig. 1.31

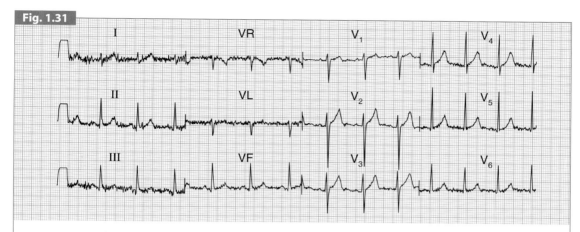

An ECG from a subject who is not relaxed
Note
- Same subject as in Figs 1.22–1.30
- The baseline is no longer clear, and is replaced by a series of sharp irregular spikes – particularly marked in the limb leads

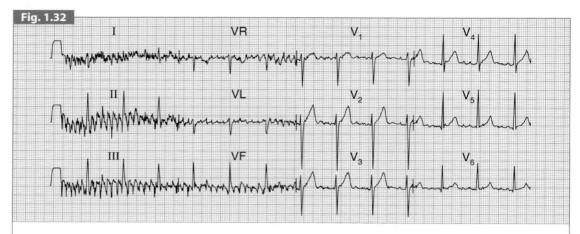

Fig. 1.32

The effect of shivering

Note

- The spikes are more exaggerated than when a patient is not relaxed
- The sharp spikes are also more synchronized, because the skeletal muscle groups are contracting together
- The effects of skeletal muscle contraction almost obliterate those of cardiac muscle contraction in leads I, II and III

HOW TO REPORT AN ECG

Many ECG recorders automatically provide a report, and in these reports the heart rate and the conducting intervals are usually accurately measured. However, the description of the rhythm and of the QRS and T patterns should be regarded with suspicion. Recorders tend to 'over-report', and to describe abnormalities where none exist: it is much better to be confident in your own reporting.

You now know enough about the ECG to understand the basis of a report. This should take the form of a description followed by an interpretation.

The description should always be given in the same sequence:

1. Rhythm
2. Conduction intervals
3. Cardiac axis
4. A description of the QRS complexes
5. A description of the ST segments and T waves.

Fig. 1.33

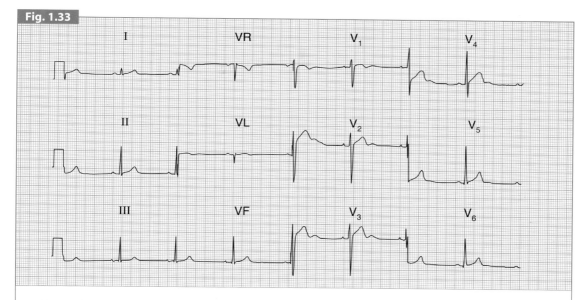

Variant of a normal ECG

Note

- Sinus rhythm, rate 50/min
- Normal PR interval (100 ms)
- Normal QRS complex duration (120 ms)
- Normal cardiac axis
- Normal QRS complexes

- Normal T waves (an inverted T wave in lead VR is normal)
- Prominent (normal) U waves in leads V_2–V_4

Interpretation

- Normal ECG

Reporting a series of totally normal findings is possibly pedantic, and in real life this is frequently not done. However, you must think about all the findings every time you interpret an ECG.

The interpretation of an ECG indicates whether the record is normal or abnormal: if abnormal, the underlying pathology needs to be identified. One of the main problems of ECG reporting is that there is quite a lot of variation in the normal ECG. Figures 1.33 and 1.34 are examples of 12-lead ECGs showing normal variants.

Fig. 1.34

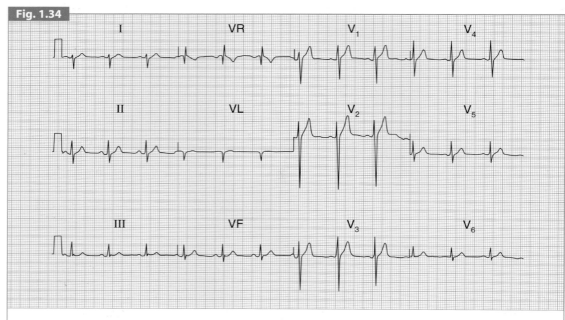

Variant of a normal ECG

Note

- Sinus rhythm, rate 75/min
- Normal PR interval (200 ms)
- Normal QRS complex duration (120 ms)
- Right axis deviation (prominent S wave in lead I)
- Normal QRS complexes
- Normal ST segments and T waves

Interpretation

- Normal ECG – apart from right axis deviation, which could be normal in a tall, thin person

REMINDERS

BASIC PRINCIPLES

- The ECG results from electrical changes associated with activation (depolarization) first of the atria and then of the ventricles.

- Atrial depolarization causes the P wave.

- Ventricular depolarization causes the QRS complex. If the first deflection is downward, it is a Q wave. Any upward deflection is an R wave. A downward deflection after an R wave is an S wave.

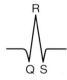

- When the depolarization wave spreads towards a lead, the deflection is predominantly upward. When the wave spreads away from a lead, the deflection is predominantly downward.

- The six limb leads (I, II, III, VR, VL and VF) look at the heart from the sides and the feet in a vertical plane.

- The cardiac axis is the average direction of spread of depolarization as seen from the front, and is estimated from leads I, II and III.

- The chest or V leads look at the heart from the front and the left side in a horizontal plane. Lead V1 is positioned over the right ventricle, and lead V6 over the left ventricle.

- The septum is depolarized from the left side to the right.

- In a normal heart the left ventricle exerts more influence on the ECG than the right ventricle.

- Unfortunately, there are a lot of minor variations in ECGs which are consistent with perfectly normal hearts. Recognizing the limits of normality is one of the main difficulties of ECG interpretation.

ECG
IP

For more on normal variants of the ECG, see Ch. 1

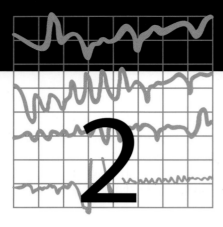

2

Conduction and its problems

We have already seen that electrical depolarization normally begins in the sinoatrial (SA) node, and that a wave of depolarization spreads outwards through the atrial muscle to the atrioventricular (AV) node, and thence down the His bundle and its branches to the ventricles. The conduction of this wave front can be delayed or blocked at any point. However, conduction problems are simple to analyse, provided you keep the wiring diagram of the heart constantly in mind (Fig. 2.1).

We can think of conduction problems in the order in which the depolarization wave normally spreads: SA node → AV node → His bundle → bundle branches. Remember in all that follows that we are assuming depolarization begins in the normal way in the SA node.

The rhythm of the heart is best interpreted from whichever ECG lead shows the P wave most clearly. This is usually, but not always, lead II or lead V_1. You can assume that all the 'rhythm strips' in this book were recorded from one of these leads.

Fig. 2.1

The wiring diagram of the heart

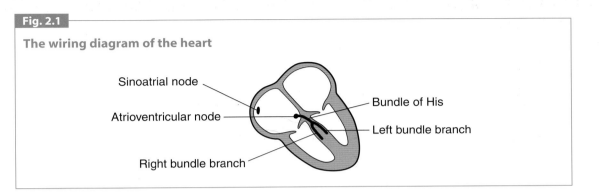

Sinoatrial node

Atrioventricular node

Right bundle branch

Bundle of His

Left bundle branch

CONDUCTION PROBLEMS IN THE AV NODE AND HIS BUNDLE

The time taken for the spread of depolarization from the SA node to the ventricular muscle is shown by the PR interval (see Ch. 1), and is not normally greater than 220 ms (six small squares).

Interference with the conduction process causes the phenomenon called 'heart block'.

PR– 0.12 – 0.20

FIRST DEGREE HEART BLOCK

If each wave of depolarization that originates in the SA node is conducted to the ventricles, but there is delay somewhere along the conduction pathway, then the PR interval is prolonged. This is called 'first degree heart block' (Fig. 2.2).

First degree heart block is not in itself important, but it may be a sign of coronary artery disease, acute rheumatic carditis, digoxin toxicity or electrolyte disturbances.

SAN – prolonged. vent.

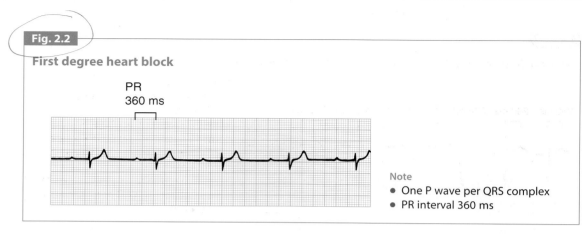

Fig. 2.2

First degree heart block

PR
360 ms

Note
- One P wave per QRS complex
- PR interval 360 ms

SECOND DEGREE HEART BLOCK

Sometimes excitation completely fails to pass through the AV node or the bundle of His. When this occurs intermittently, 'second degree heart block' is said to exist. There are three variations of this:

1. There may be progressive lengthening of the PR interval and then failure of conduction of an atrial beat, followed by a conducted beat with a shorter PR interval and then a repetition of this cycle. This is the 'Wenckebach' or 'Mobitz type 1' phenomenon (Fig. 2.3).
2. Most beats are conducted with a constant PR interval, but occasionally there is atrial depolarization without a subsequent ventricular depolarization. This is called the 'Mobitz type 2' phenomenon (Fig. 2.4).
3. There may be alternate conducted and nonconducted atrial beats (or one conducted atrial beat and then two or three nonconducted beats), giving twice (or three or four times) as many P waves as QRS complexes. This is called '2:1' ('two to one'), '3:1' ('three to one') or '4:1' ('four to one') conduction (Fig. 2.5).

It is important to remember that, as with any other rhythm, a P wave may only show itself as a distortion of a T wave (Fig. 2.6).

Fig. 2.3

Second degree heart block (Wenckebach (Mobitz type 1))

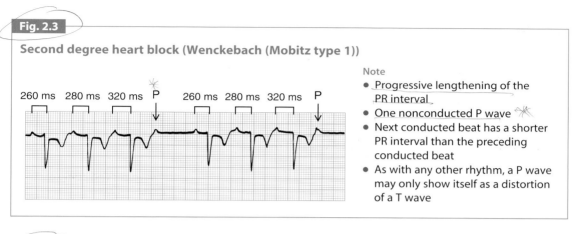

260 ms   280 ms   320 ms   P   260 ms   280 ms   320 ms   P

Note

- Progressive lengthening of the PR interval
- One nonconducted P wave
- Next conducted beat has a shorter PR interval than the preceding conducted beat
- As with any other rhythm, a P wave may only show itself as a distortion of a T wave

Fig. 2.4

Second degree heart block (Mobitz type 2)

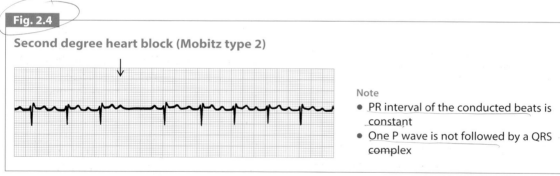

Note

- PR interval of the conducted beats is constant
- One P wave is not followed by a QRS complex

The underlying causes of second degree heart block are the same as those of first degree block. The Wenckebach phenomenon is usually benign, but Mobitz type 2 block and 2:1, 3:1 or 4:1 block may herald 'complete,' or 'third degree', heart block.

Fig. 2.5

Second degree heart block (2:1 type)

P

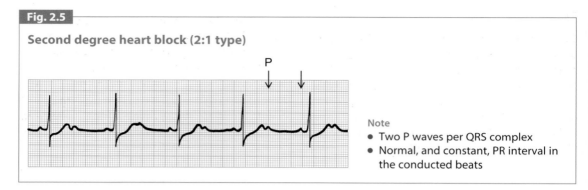

Note
- Two P waves per QRS complex
- Normal, and constant, PR interval in the conducted beats

Fig. 2.6

Second degree heart block (2:1 type)

P

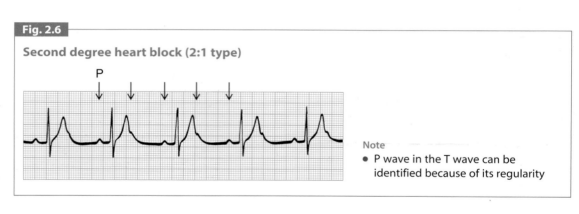

Note
- P wave in the T wave can be identified because of its regularity

THIRD DEGREE HEART BLOCK

Complete heart block (third degree block) is said to occur when atrial contraction is normal but no beats are conducted to the ventricles (Fig. 2.7). When this occurs the ventricles are excited by a slow 'escape mechanism' (see Ch. 3), from a depolarizing focus within the ventricular muscle.

Complete block is not always immediately obvious in a 12-lead ECG, where there may be only a few QRS complexes per lead (e.g. see Fig. 2.8). You have to look at the PR interval in all the leads to see that there is no consistency.

Complete heart block may occur as an acute phenomenon in patients with myocardial infarction (when it is usually transient) or it may be chronic, usually due to fibrosis around the bundle of His. It may also be caused by the block of both bundle branches.

Fig. 2.7

Third degree heart block

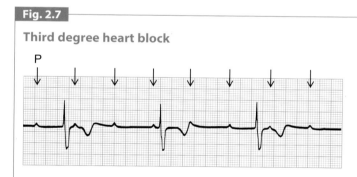

Note
- P wave rate 90/min
- No relationship between P waves and QRS complexes
- QRS complex rate 36/min
- Abnormally shaped QRS complexes, because of abnormal spread of depolarization from a ventricular focus

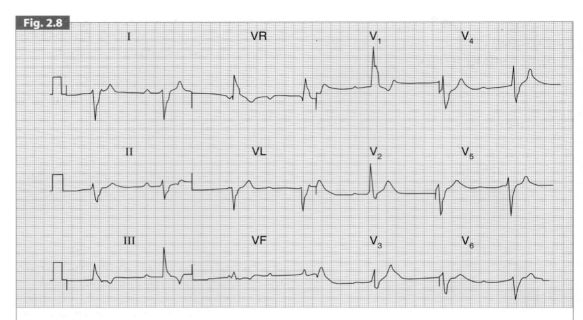

Fig. 2.8

Complete heart block

Note

- Sinus rhythm, but no P waves are conducted
- Right axis deviation
- Broad QRS complexes (duration 160 ms)
- Right bundle branch block pattern

- In this case the cause of the block could not be determined, though in most patients it results from fibrosis of the bundle of His

CONDUCTION PROBLEMS IN THE RIGHT AND LEFT BUNDLE BRANCHES – BUNDLE BRANCH BLOCK

If the depolarization wave reaches the interventricular septum normally, the interval between the beginning of the P wave and the first deflection in the QRS complex (the PR interval) will be normal. However, if there is abnormal conduction through either the right or left bundle branches ('bundle branch block') there will be a delay in the depolarization of part of the ventricular muscle. The extra time taken for depolarization of the whole of the ventricular muscle causes widening of the QRS complex.

In the normal heart, the time taken for the depolarization wave to spread from the interventricular septum to the furthest part of the ventricles is less than 120 ms, represented by three small squares of ECG paper. If the QRS complex duration is greater than 120 ms, then conduction within the ventricles must have occurred by an abnormal, and therefore slower, pathway.

A wide QRS complex can therefore indicate bundle branch block, but widening also occurs if depolarization begins within the ventricular muscle itself (see Ch. 3). However, remember that in sinus rhythm with bundle branch block, normal P waves are present with a constant PR interval. We shall see that this is not the case with rhythms beginning in the ventricles.

Block of both bundle branches has the same effect as block of the His bundle, and causes complete (third degree) heart block.

Right bundle branch block (RBBB) often indicates problems in the right side of the heart, but RBBB patterns with a QRS complex of normal duration are quite common in healthy people.

Left bundle branch block (LBBB) is always an indication of heart disease, usually of the left ventricle.

It is important to recognize when bundle branch block is present, because LBBB prevents any further interpretation of the cardiogram, and RBBB can make interpretation difficult.

The mechanism underlying the ECG patterns of RBBB and LBBB can be worked out from first principles. Remember (see Ch. 1):

- The septum is normally depolarized from left to right.
- The left ventricle, having the greater muscle mass, exerts more influence on the ECG than does the right ventricle.
- Excitation spreading towards a lead causes an upward deflection within the ECG.

RIGHT BUNDLE BRANCH BLOCK

In RBBB, no conduction occurs down the right bundle branch but the septum is depolarized from the left side as usual, causing an R wave in a right ventricular lead (V_1) and a small Q wave in a left ventricular lead (V_6) (Fig. 2.9).

Excitation then spreads to the left ventricle, causing an S wave in lead V_1 and an R wave in lead V_6 (Fig. 2.10).

It takes longer than in a normal heart for excitation to reach the right ventricle because of the failure of the normal conducting pathway. The right ventricle therefore depolarizes after the left. This causes a second R wave (R^1) in lead V_1, and a wide and deep S wave, and consequently a wide QRS complex, in lead V_6 (Fig. 2.11).

An 'RSR^1' pattern, with a QRS complex of normal width (less than 120 ms), is sometimes called 'partial right bundle branch block'. It is seldom of significance, and can be considered to be a normal variant.

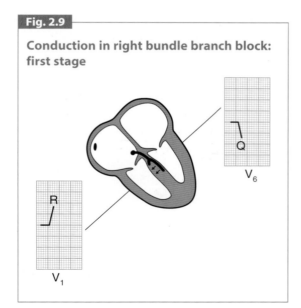

Fig. 2.9

Conduction in right bundle branch block: first stage

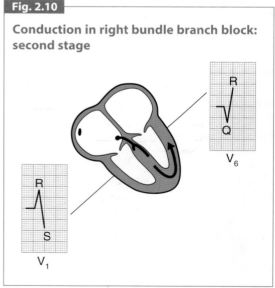

Fig. 2.10

Conduction in right bundle branch block: second stage

LEFT BUNDLE BRANCH BLOCK

If conduction down the left bundle branch fails, the septum becomes depolarized from right to left, causing a small Q wave in lead V_1, and an R wave in lead V_6 (Fig. 2.12).

The right ventricle is depolarized before the left, so despite the smaller muscle mass there is an R wave in lead V_1 and an S wave (often appearing only as a notch) in lead V_6 (Fig. 2.13). Remember that any upward deflection, however small, is an R wave, and any downward deflection, however small, following an R wave is called an S wave.

Subsequent depolarization of the left ventricle causes an S wave in lead V_1 and another R wave in lead V_6 (Fig. 2.14).

LBBB is associated with T wave inversion in the lateral leads (I, VL and V_5–V_6), though not necessarily in all of these.

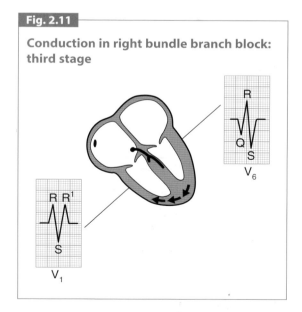

Fig. 2.11

Conduction in right bundle branch block: third stage

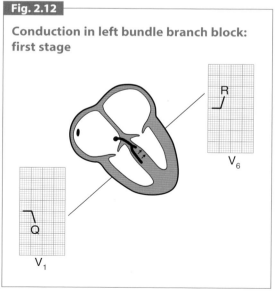

Fig. 2.12

Conduction in left bundle branch block: first stage

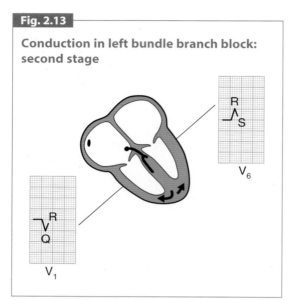

Fig. 2.13

Conduction in left bundle branch block: second stage

V_6

V_1

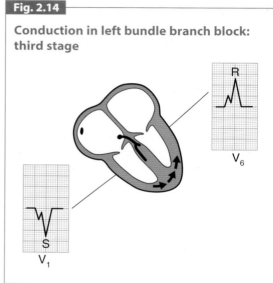

Fig. 2.14

Conduction in left bundle branch block: third stage

V_6

V_1

REMINDERS

BUNDLE BRANCH BLOCK

- RBBB is best seen in lead V_1, where there is an RSR[1] pattern (Fig. 2.15).
- LBBB is best seen in lead V_6, where there is a broad QRS complex with a notched top, which resembles the letter 'M' and is therefore known as an 'M' pattern (Fig. 2.16). The complete picture, with a 'W' pattern in lead V_1, is often not fully developed.

Fig. 2.15

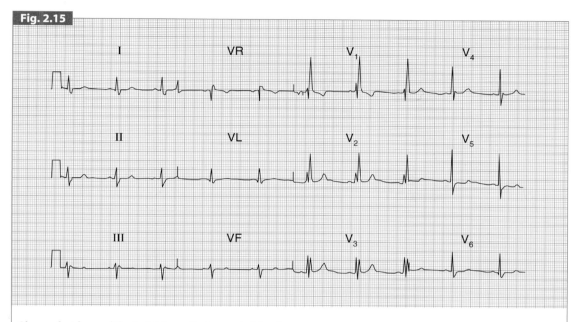

Sinus rhythm with right bundle branch block

Note

- Sinus rhythm, rate 60/min
- Normal PR interval
- Normal cardiac axis
- Wide QRS complexes (160 ms)
- RSR[1] pattern in lead V_1 and deep, wide S waves in lead V_6
- Normal ST segments and T waves

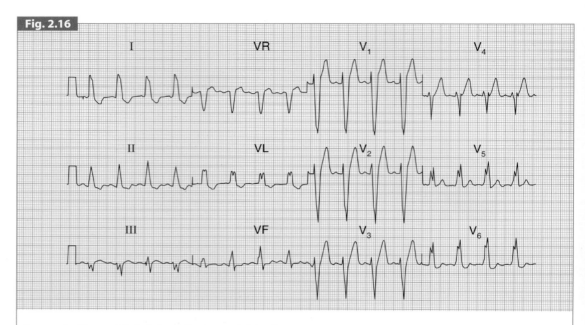

Fig. 2.16

Sinus rhythm with left bundle branch block

Note

- Sinus rhythm, rate 100/min
- Normal PR interval
- Normal cardiac axis
- Wide QRS complexes (160 ms)
- M pattern in the QRS complexes, best seen in leads I, VL, V$_5$ and V$_6$
- Inverted T waves in leads I, II, VL

CONDUCTION PROBLEMS IN THE DISTAL PARTS OF THE LEFT BUNDLE BRANCH

At this point it is worth considering in a little more detail the anatomy of the branches of the His bundle. The right bundle branch has no main divisions, but the left bundle branch has two – the anterior and posterior 'fascicles'. The depolarization wave therefore spreads into the ventricles by three pathways (Fig. 2.17).

The cardiac axis (see Ch. 1) depends on the average direction of depolarization of the ventricles. Because the left ventricle contains more muscle than the right, it has more influence on the cardiac axis (Fig. 2.18).

If the anterior fascicle of the left bundle branch fails to conduct, the left ventricle has to be depolarized through the posterior fascicle, and so the cardiac axis rotates upwards (Fig. 2.19).

Left axis deviation is therefore due to left anterior fascicular block, or 'left anterior hemiblock' (Fig. 2.20).

Fig. 2.17

The three pathways of the depolarization wave

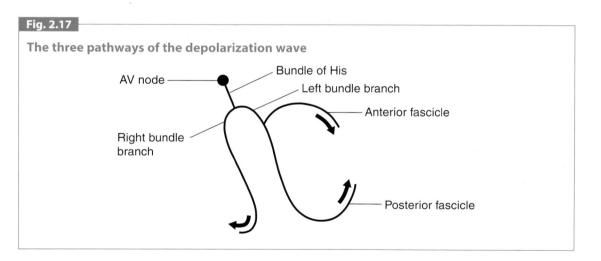

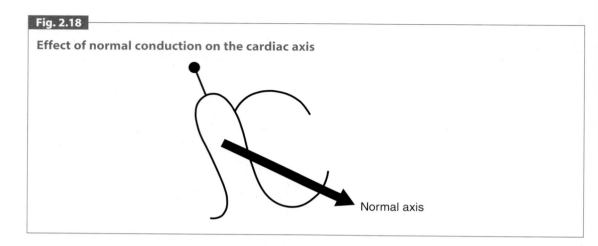

Fig. 2.18

Effect of normal conduction on the cardiac axis

Normal axis

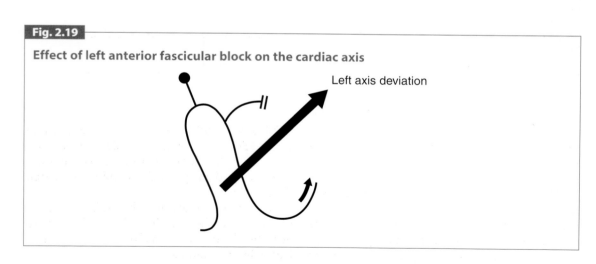

Fig. 2.19

Effect of left anterior fascicular block on the cardiac axis

Left axis deviation

Fig. 2.20

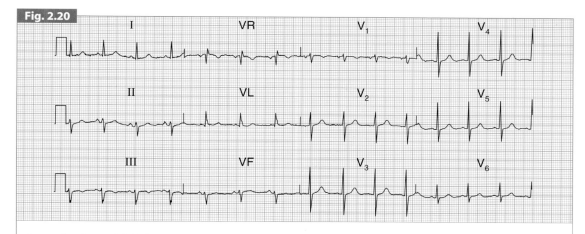

Sinus rhythm with left axis deviation (otherwise normal)

Note

- Sinus rhythm, rate 80/min
- Left axis deviation: QRS complex upright in lead I, but downward (dominant S wave) in leads II and III
- Normal QRS complexes, ST segments and T waves

The posterior fascicle of the left bundle is only rarely selectively blocked, in 'left posterior hemiblock', but if this does occur the ECG shows right axis deviation.

When the right bundle branch is blocked, the cardiac axis usually remains normal, because there is normal depolarization of the left ventricle with its large muscle mass (Fig. 2.21).

However, if both the right bundle branch and the left anterior fascicle are blocked, the ECG shows RBBB and left axis deviation (Fig. 2.22). This is sometimes called 'bifascicular block', and this ECG pattern obviously indicates widespread damage to the conducting system (Fig. 2.23).

If the right bundle branch and both fascicles of the left bundle branch are blocked, complete heart block occurs just as if the main His bundle had failed to conduct.

Fig. 2.21

Lack of effect of right bundle branch block on the cardiac axis

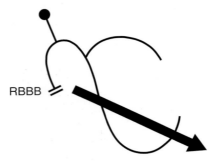

RBBB

Fig. 2.22

Effect of right bundle branch block and left anterior hemiblock on the cardiac axis

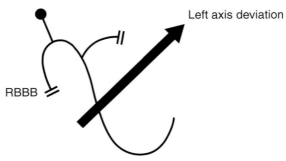

Left axis deviation

RBBB

Fig. 2.23

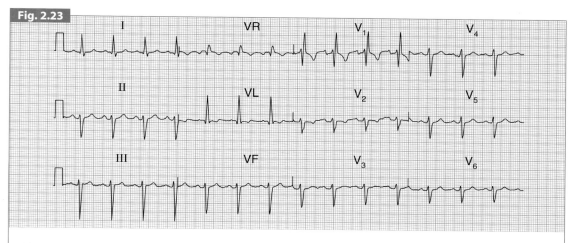

Bifascicular block

Note

- Sinus rhythm, rate 90/min
- Left axis deviation (dominant S wave in leads II and III)
- Right bundle branch block (RSR[1] pattern in lead V_1, and deep, wide S wave in lead V_6)

WHAT TO DO

Always remember that it is the patient who should be treated, not the ECG. Relief of symptoms always comes first. However, some general points can be made about the action that might be taken if the ECG shows conduction abnormalities.

First degree block

- Often seen in normal people.
- Think about acute myocardial infarction and acute rheumatic fever as possible causes.
- No specific action needed.

Second degree block

- Usually indicates heart disease; often seen in acute myocardial infarction.
- Mobitz type 2 and Wenckebach block do not need specific treatment.
- 2:1, 3:1 or 4:1 block may indicate a need for temporary or permanent pacing, especially if the ventricular rate is slow.

Third degree block

- Always indicates conducting tissue disease – more often fibrosis than ischaemic.
- Consider a temporary or permanent pacemaker.

Right bundle branch block

- Think about an atrial septal defect.
- No specific treatment.

Left bundle branch block

- Think about aortic stenosis and ischaemic disease.
- If the patient is asymptomatic, no action is needed.
- If the patient has recently had severe chest pain, LBBB may indicate an acute myocardial infarction, and intervention should be considered.

Left axis deviation

- Think about left ventricular hypertrophy and its causes.
- No action needed.

Left axis deviation and right bundle branch block

- Indicates severe conducting tissue disease.
- No specific treatment needed.
- Pacemaker required if the patient has symptoms suggestive of intermittent complete heart block.

REMINDERS

CONDUCTION AND ITS EFFECTS ON THE ECG

- Depolarization normally begins in the SA node, and spreads to the ventricles via the AV node, the His bundle, the right and left branches of the His bundle, and the anterior and posterior fascicles of the left bundle branch.

- A conduction abnormality can develop at any of these points.

- Conduction problems in the AV node and His bundle may be partial (first and second degree block) or complete (third degree block).

- If conduction is normal through the AV node, the His bundle and one of its branches, but is abnormal in the other branch, bundle branch block exists and the QRS complex is wide.

- The ECG pattern of RBBB and LBBB can be worked out if you remember that:
  - the septum is depolarized first from left to right
  - lead V_1 looks at the right ventricle and lead V_6 at the left ventricle
  - when depolarization spreads towards an electrode the stylus moves upwards.

- If you can't remember all this, remember that RBBB has an RSR[1] pattern in lead V_1, while LBBB has a letter 'M' pattern in lead V_6.

- Block of the anterior division or fascicle of the left bundle branch causes left axis deviation.

For more on conduction problems, see pp. 85–95

For more on treatment of conduction problems with pacemakers, see pp. 187–206

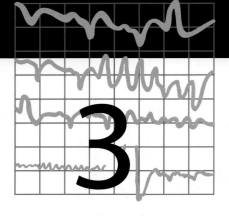

3

The rhythm of the heart

So far we have only considered the spread of depolarization that follows the normal activation of the sinoatrial (SA) node. When depolarization begins in the SA node the heart is said to be in sinus rhythm. Depolarization can, however, begin in other places. Then the rhythm is named after the part of the heart where the depolarization sequence originates, and an 'arrhythmia' is said to be present.

When attempting to analyse a cardiac rhythm remember:

- Atrial contraction is associated with the P wave of the ECG.
- Ventricular contraction is associated with the QRS complex.
- Atrial contraction normally precedes ventricular contraction, and there is normally one atrial contraction per ventricular contraction (i.e. there should be as many P waves as there are QRS complexes).

The keys to rhythm abnormalities are:

- The P waves – can you find them? Look for the lead in which they are most obvious.
- The relationship between the P waves and the QRS complexes – there should be one P wave per QRS complex.

- The width of the QRS complexes (should be 120 ms or less).
- Because an arrhythmia should be identified from the lead in which the P waves can be seen most easily, full 12-lead ECGs are better than rhythm strips.

THE INTRINSIC RHYTHMICITY OF THE HEART

Most parts of the heart can depolarize spontaneously and rhythmically, and the rate of contraction of the ventricles will be controlled by the part of the heart that is depolarizing most frequently.

The stars in the figures in this chapter indicate the part of the heart where the activation sequence began. The SA node normally has the highest frequency of discharge. Therefore the rate of contraction of the ventricles will equal the rate of discharge of the SA node. The rate of discharge of the SA node is influenced by the vagus nerves, and also by reflexes originating in the lungs. Changes in heart rate associated with respiration are normally seen in young people, and this is called 'sinus arrhythmia' (Fig. 3.1).

A slow sinus rhythm ('sinus bradycardia') can be associated with athletic training, fainting attacks, hypothermia or myxoedema, and is also often seen immediately after a heart attack. A fast sinus rhythm ('sinus tachycardia') can be associated with exercise, fear, pain, haemorrhage or thyrotoxicosis. There is no particular rate that is called 'bradycardia' or 'tachycardia' – these are merely descriptive terms.

Fig. 3.1

Sinus arrhythmia

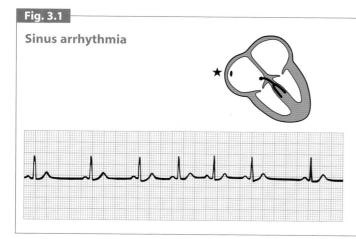

Note
- One P wave per QRS complex
- Constant PR interval
- Progressive beat-to-beat change in the R–R interval

ABNORMAL RHYTHMS

Abnormal cardiac rhythms can begin in one of three places (Fig. 3.2): the atrial muscle; the region around the atrioventricular (AV) node (this is called 'nodal' or, more properly, junctional'); or the ventricular muscle. Although

Figure 3.2 suggests that electrical activation might begin at specific points within the atrial and ventricular muscles, abnormal rhythms can begin anywhere within the atria or ventricles.

Sinus rhythm, atrial rhythm and junctional rhythm together constitute the 'supraventricular' rhythms (Fig. 3.3). In the supraventricular

Fig. 3.2

Points where cardiac rhythms can begin

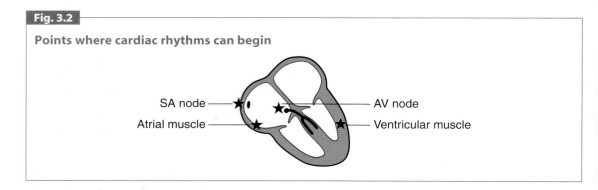

Fig. 3.3

Division of abnormal rhythms into supraventricular and ventricular

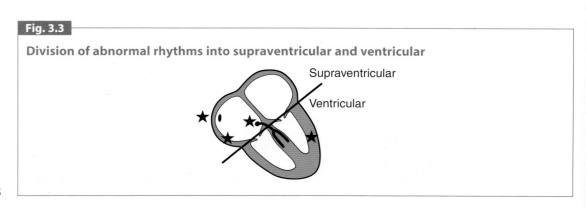

rhythms, the depolarization wave spreads to the ventricles in the normal way via the His bundle and its branches (Fig. 3.4). The QRS complex is therefore normal, and is the same whether depolarization was initiated by

the SA node, the atrial muscle, or the junctional region.

In ventricular rhythms, on the other hand, the depolarization wave spreads through the ventricles by an abnormal and slower pathway, via the Purkinje fibres (Fig. 3.5). The QRS complex is therefore wide and is abnormally shaped. Repolarization is also abnormal, so the T wave is also of abnormal shape.

Remember:

- Supraventricular rhythms have narrow QRS complexes.
- Ventricular rhythms have wide QRS complexes.
- The only exception to this rule occurs when there is a supraventricular rhythm with right or left bundle branch block, or the Wolff–Parkinson–White (WPW) syndrome, when the QRS complex will be wide (see p. 79).

Abnormal rhythms arising in the atrial muscle, the junctional region or the ventricular muscle can be categorized as:

- bradycardias – slow and sustained
- extrasystoles – occur as early single beats
- tachycardias – fast and sustained
- fibrillation – activation of the atria or ventricles is totally disorganized.

THE BRADYCARDIAS – THE SLOW RHYTHMS

It is clearly advantageous if different parts of the heart are able to initiate the depolarization **59**

Fig. 3.4

Spread of the depolarization wave in supraventricular rhythms

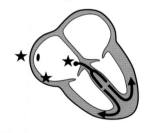

Fig. 3.5

Spread of the depolarization wave in ventricular rhythm

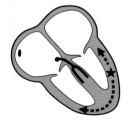

sequence, because this gives the heart a series of failsafe mechanisms that will keep it going if the SA node fails to depolarize, or if conduction of the depolarization wave is blocked. However, the protective mechanisms must normally be inactive if competition between normal and abnormal sites of spontaneous depolarization is to be avoided. This is achieved by the secondary sites having a lower intrinsic frequency of depolarization than the SA node.

The heart is controlled by whichever site is spontaneously depolarizing most frequently: normally this is the SA node, and it gives a normal heart rate of about 70/min. If the SA node fails to depolarize, control will be assumed by a focus either in the atrial muscle or in the region around the AV node (the junctional region), both of which have spontaneous depolarization frequencies of about 50/min. If these fail, or if conduction through the His bundle is blocked, a ventricular focus will take over and give a ventricular rate of about 30/min.

These slow and protective rhythms are called 'escape rhythms', because they occur when secondary sites for initiating depolarization escape from their normal inhibition by the more active SA node.

Escape rhythms are not primary disorders, but are the response to problems higher in the conducting pathway. They are commonly seen in the acute phase of a heart attack, when they may be associated with sinus bradycardia. It is important not to try to suppress an escape rhythm, because without it the heart might stop altogether.

ATRIAL ESCAPE

If the rate of depolarization of the SA node slows down and a different focus in the atrium takes over control of the heart, the rhythm is described as 'atrial escape' (Fig. 3.6). Atrial escape beats can occur singly.

NODAL (JUNCTIONAL) ESCAPE

If the region around the AV node takes over as the focus of depolarization, the rhythm is called 'nodal', or more properly, 'junctional' escape (Fig. 3.7).

VENTRICULAR ESCAPE

'Ventricular escape' is most commonly seen when conduction between the atria and ventricles is interrupted by complete heart block (Fig. 3.8).

Ventricular escape rhythms can occur without complete heart block, and ventricular escape beats can be single (Fig. 3.9).

The rhythm of the heart can occasionally be controlled by a ventricular focus with an intrinsic frequency of discharge faster than that seen in complete heart block. This rhythm is called 'accelerated idioventricular rhythm' (Fig. 3.10), and is often associated with acute myocardial infarction. Although the appearance of the ECG is similar to that of ventricular tachycardia (described later), accelerated idioventricular rhythm is benign and should not be treated. Ventricular tachycardia should not be diagnosed unless the heart rate exceeds 120/min.

Fig. 3.6

Atrial escape

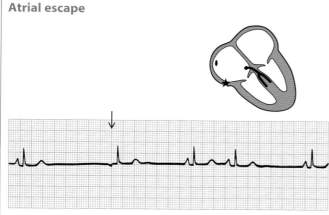

Note

- After one sinus beat the SA node fails to depolarize
- After a delay, an abnormal P wave is seen because excitation of the atrium has begun somewhere other than the SA node
- The abnormal P wave is followed by a normal QRS complex, because excitation has spread normally down the His bundle
- The remaining beats show a return to sinus arrhythmia

Fig. 3.7

Nodal (junctional) escape

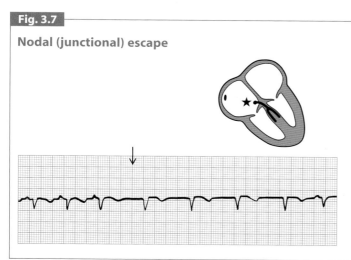

Note

- Sinus rhythm, rate 100/min
- Junctional escape rhythm (following the arrow), rate 75/min
- No P waves in junctional beats (indicates either no atrial contraction or P wave lost in QRS complex)
- Normal QRS complexes

Fig. 3.8

Complete heart block

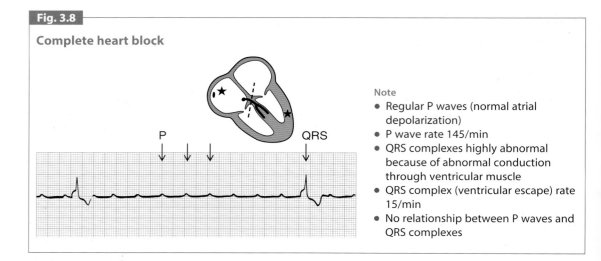

P   QRS

Note
- Regular P waves (normal atrial depolarization)
- P wave rate 145/min
- QRS complexes highly abnormal because of abnormal conduction through ventricular muscle
- QRS complex (ventricular escape) rate 15/min
- No relationship between P waves and QRS complexes

Fig. 3.9

Ventricular escape

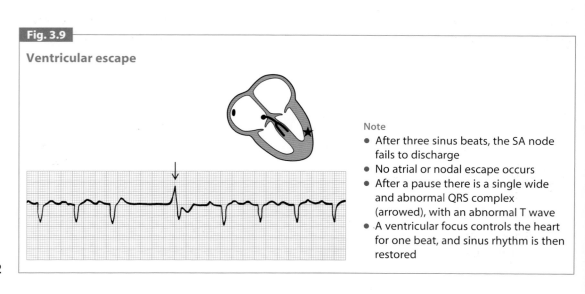

Note
- After three sinus beats, the SA node fails to discharge
- No atrial or nodal escape occurs
- After a pause there is a single wide and abnormal QRS complex (arrowed), with an abnormal T wave
- A ventricular focus controls the heart for one beat, and sinus rhythm is then restored

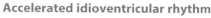

Fig. 3.10

Accelerated idioventricular rhythm

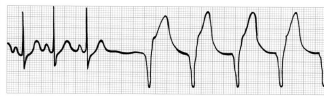

Note
- After three sinus beats, the SA node fails to depolarize
- An escape focus in the ventricle takes over, causing a regular rhythm of 75/min with wide QRS complexes and abnormal T waves

EXTRASYSTOLES

Any part of the heart can depolarize earlier than it should, and the accompanying heartbeat is called an extrasystole. The term 'ectopic' is sometimes used to indicate that depolarization originated in an abnormal location, and the term 'premature contraction' means the same thing.

The ECG appearance of an extrasystole arising in the atrial muscle, the junctional or nodal region, or the ventricular muscle, is the same as that of the corresponding escape beat – the difference is that an extrasystole comes early and an escape beat comes late.

Atrial extrasystoles have abnormal P waves (Fig. 3.11). In a junctional extrasystole there is

Fig. 3.11

Atrial and junctional (nodal) extrasystoles

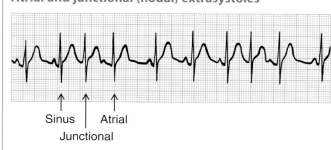

Sinus | Atrial
Junctional

Note
- This record shows sinus rhythm with junctional and atrial extrasystoles
- A junctional extrasystole has no P wave
- An atrial extrasystole has an abnormally shaped P wave
- Sinus, junctional and atrial beats have identical QRS complexes – conduction in and beyond the His bundle is normal

no P wave at all, or the P wave appears immediately before or immediately after the QRS complex (Fig. 3.11). The QRS complexes of atrial and junctional extrasystoles are, of course, the same as those of sinus rhythm.

Ventricular extrasystoles, however, have abnormal QRS complexes, which are typically wide and can be of almost any shape (Fig. 3.12).

Ventricular extrasystoles are common, and are usually of no importance. However, when they occur early in the T wave of a preceding beat they can induce ventricular fibrillation (see p. 79), and are thus potentially dangerous.

It may, however, not be as easy as this, particularly if a beat of supraventricular origin is conducted abnormally to the ventricles

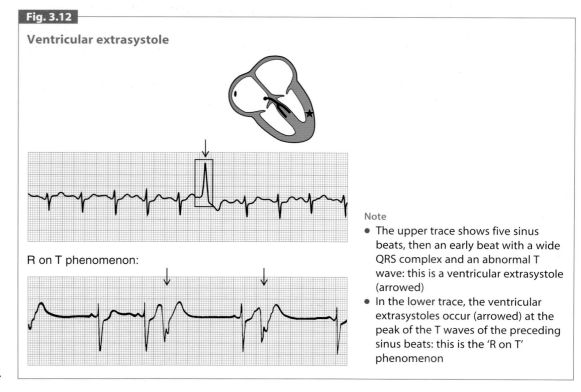

Fig. 3.12

Ventricular extrasystole

R on T phenomenon:

Note
- The upper trace shows five sinus beats, then an early beat with a wide QRS complex and an abnormal T wave: this is a ventricular extrasystole (arrowed)
- In the lower trace, the ventricular extrasystoles occur (arrowed) at the peak of the T waves of the preceding sinus beats: this is the 'R on T' phenomenon

(bundle branch block, see Ch. 2). It is advisable to get into the habit of asking five questions every time an ECG is being analysed:

1. Does an early QRS complex follow an early P wave? If so, it must be an atrial extrasystole.
2. Can a P wave be seen anywhere? A junctional extrasystole may cause the appearance of a P wave very close to, and even after, the QRS complex because excitation is conducted both to the atria and to the ventricles.
3. Is the QRS complex the same shape throughout (i.e. has it the same initial direction of deflection as the normal beat, and has it the same duration)? Supraventricular beats look the same as each other; ventricular beats may look different from each other.
4. Is the T wave the same way up as in the normal beat? In supraventricular beats, it is the same way up; in ventricular beats, it is inverted.
5. Does the next P wave after the extrasystole appear at an expected time? In both supraventricular and ventricular extrasystoles there is a ('compensatory') pause before the next heartbeat, but a supraventricular extrasystole usually upsets the normal periodicity of the SA node, so that the next SA node discharge (and P wave) comes late.

The effects of both supraventricular and ventricular extrasystoles on the following P wave are as follows:

- A supraventricular extrasystole resets the P wave cycle (Fig. 3.13).

Fig. 3.13

Supraventricular extrasystole

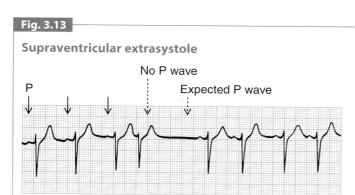

No P wave

P

Expected P wave

Note
- Three sinus beats are followed by a junctional extrasystole
- No P wave is seen at the expected time, and the next P wave is late

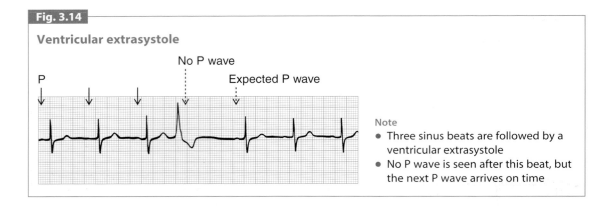

Fig. 3.14

Ventricular extrasystole

No P wave

P

Expected P wave

Note
- Three sinus beats are followed by a ventricular extrasystole
- No P wave is seen after this beat, but the next P wave arrives on time

- A ventricular extrasystole, on the other hand, does not affect the SA node, so the next P wave appears at the predicted time (Fig. 3.14).

THE TACHYCARDIAS – THE FAST RHYTHMS

Foci in the atria, the junctional (AV nodal) region, and the ventricles may depolarize repeatedly, causing a sustained tachycardia. The criteria already described can be used to decide the origin of the arrhythmia, and as before the most important thing is to try to identify a P wave. When a tachycardia occurs intermittently, it is called 'paroxysmal': this is a clinical description, and is not related to any specific ECG pattern.

SUPRAVENTRICULAR TACHYCARDIAS

Atrial tachycardia (abnormal focus in the atrium)

In atrial tachycardia, the atria depolarize faster than 150/min (Fig. 3.15).

The AV node cannot conduct atrial rates of discharge greater than about 200/min. If the atrial rate is faster than this, 'atrioventricular block' occurs, with some P waves not followed by QRS complexes. The difference between this sort of atrioventricular block and second degree heart block is that in atrioventricular block

---

Fig. 3.15

Atrial tachycardia

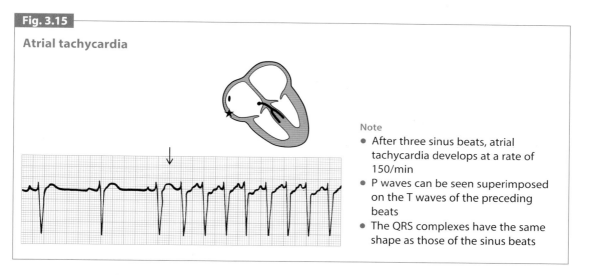

Note
- After three sinus beats, atrial tachycardia develops at a rate of 150/min
- P waves can be seen superimposed on the T waves of the preceding beats
- The QRS complexes have the same shape as those of the sinus beats

---

associated with tachycardia the AV node is functioning properly – it is preventing the ventricles from being activated at a fast (and therefore inefficient) rate. In first, second or third degree block associated with sinus rhythm, the AV node and/or the His bundle are not conducting normally.

Atrial flutter

When the atrial rate is greater than 250/min, and there is no flat baseline between the P waves, 'atrial flutter' is present (Fig. 3.16).

When atrial tachycardia or atrial flutter is associated with 2:1 block, you need to look carefully to recognize the extra P waves (Fig. 3.17). A narrow complex tachycardia with a ventricular rate of about 125–150/min should always alert you to the possibility of atrial flutter with 2:1 block.

Any arrhythmia should be identified from the lead in which P waves can most easily be seen. In the record in Figure 3.18, atrial flutter is most easily seen in lead II, but it is also obvious in leads VR and VF.

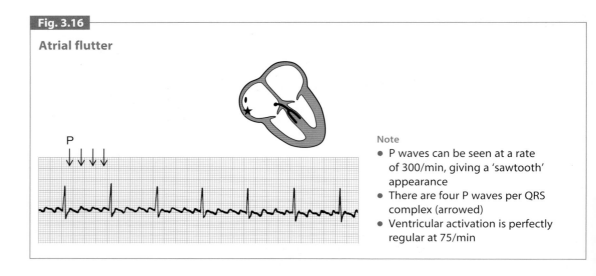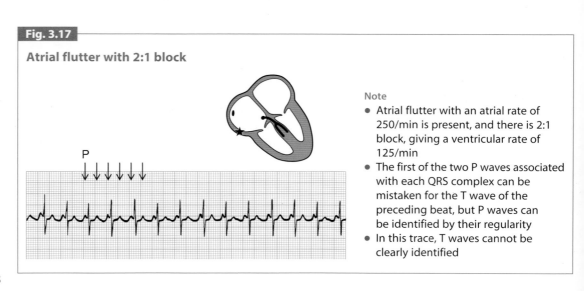

Fig. 3.16

Atrial flutter

Note
- P waves can be seen at a rate of 300/min, giving a 'sawtooth' appearance
- There are four P waves per QRS complex (arrowed)
- Ventricular activation is perfectly regular at 75/min

Fig. 3.17

Atrial flutter with 2:1 block

Note
- Atrial flutter with an atrial rate of 250/min is present, and there is 2:1 block, giving a ventricular rate of 125/min
- The first of the two P waves associated with each QRS complex can be mistaken for the T wave of the preceding beat, but P waves can be identified by their regularity
- In this trace, T waves cannot be clearly identified

Fig. 3.18

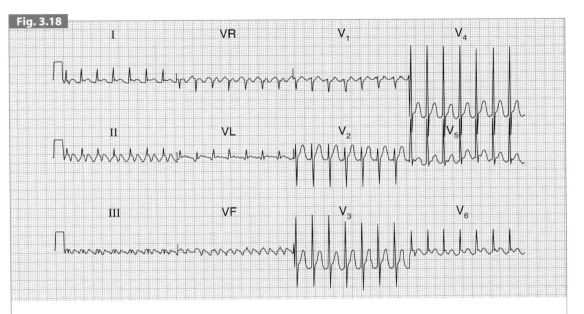

Atrial flutter with 2:1 block

Note
- P waves at just over 300/min (most easily seen in leads II and VR)
- Regular QRS complexes, rate 160/min
- Narrow QRS complexes of normal shape
- Normal T waves (best seen in the V leads; in the limb leads it is difficult to distinguish between T and P waves)

Junctional (nodal) tachycardia

If the area around the AV node depolarizes frequently, the P waves may be seen very close to the QRS complexes, or may not be seen at all (Fig. 3.19). The QRS complex is of normal shape because, as with the other supraventricular arrhythmias, the ventricles are activated via the His bundle in the normal way.

The 12-lead ECG in Figure 3.20 shows that in junctional tachycardia no P waves can be seen in any lead.

Fig. 3.19

Junctional (nodal) tachycardia

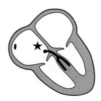

Junctional tachycardia:

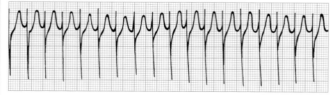

Sinus rhythm:

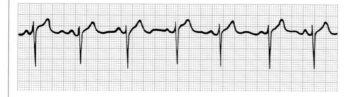

Note
- In the upper trace there are no P waves, and the QRS complexes are completely regular
- The lower trace is from the same patient, in sinus rhythm. The QRS complexes have essentially the same shape as those of the junctional tachycardia

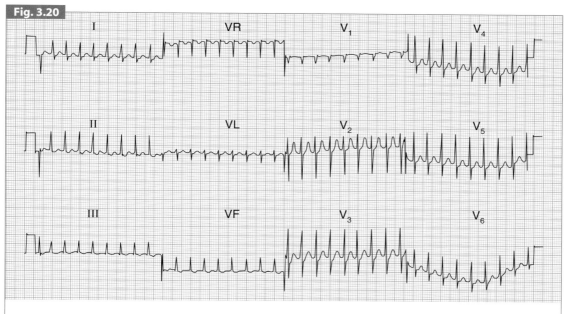

Fig. 3.20

Junctional tachycardia

Note

- No P waves
- Regular QRS complexes, rate 200/min
- Narrow QRS complexes of normal shape
- Normal T waves

Carotid sinus pressure

Carotid sinus pressure may have a useful therapeutic effect on supraventricular tachycardias, and is always worth trying because it may make the nature of the arrhythmia more obvious (Fig. 3.21). Carotid sinus pressure activates a reflex that leads to vagal stimulation of the SA and AV nodes. This causes a reduction in the frequency of discharge of the SA node, and an increase in the delay of conduction in the AV node. It is the latter which is important in the diagnosis and treatment of arrhythmias. Carotid sinus pressure completely abolishes some supraventricular arrhythmias, and slows the ventricular rate in others, but it has no effect on ventricular arrhythmias.

Fig. 3.21

Atrial flutter with carotid sinus pressure (CSP)

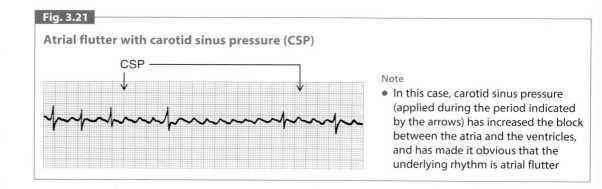

CSP

Note
- In this case, carotid sinus pressure (applied during the period indicated by the arrows) has increased the block between the atria and the ventricles, and has made it obvious that the underlying rhythm is atrial flutter

VENTRICULAR TACHYCARDIAS

If a focus in the ventricular muscle depolarizes with a high frequency (causing, in effect, rapidly repeated ventricular extrasystoles), the rhythm is called 'ventricular tachycardia' (Fig. 3.22).

Excitation has to spread by an abnormal path through the ventricular muscle, and the QRS complex is therefore wide and abnormal.

Wide and abnormal complexes are seen in all 12 leads of the standard ECG (Fig. 3.23).

Remember that wide and abnormal complexes are also seen with bundle branch block (Fig. 3.24).

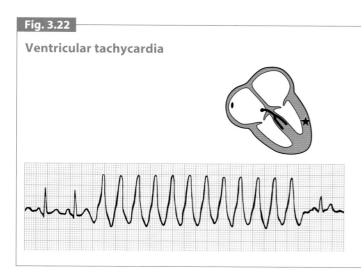

Fig. 3.22

Ventricular tachycardia

Note
- After two sinus beats, the rate increases to 200/min
- The QRS complexes become broad, and the T waves are difficult to identify
- The final beat shows a return to sinus rhythm

ECG
IP

For more on broad complex tachycardias, see p. 126

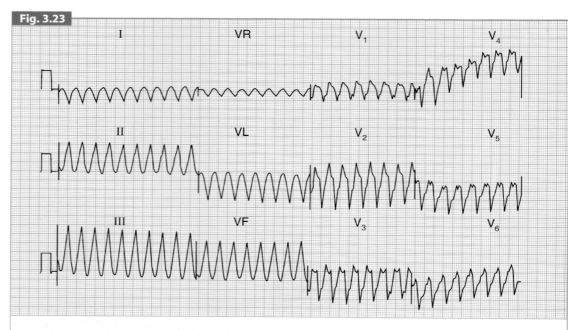

Fig. 3.23

Ventricular tachycardia

Note
- No P waves
- Regular QRS complexes, rate 200/min
- Broad QRS complexes, duration 280 ms, with a very abnormal shape
- No identifiable T waves

| Fig. 3.24 |

Sinus rhythm with left bundle branch block

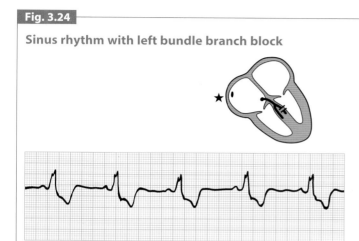

Note

- Sinus rhythm: each QRS complex is preceded by a P wave, with a constant PR interval
- The QRS complexes are wide and the T waves are inverted
- This trace was recorded from lead V_6, and the M pattern and inverted T wave characteristic of left bundle branch block are easily identifiable

HOW TO DISTINGUISH BETWEEN VENTRICULAR TACHYCARDIA AND SUPRAVENTRICULAR TACHYCARDIA WITH BUNDLE BRANCH BLOCK

It is essential to remember that the patient's clinical state – whether good or bad – does not help to differentiate between the two possible causes of a tachycardia with broad QRS complexes. If a patient with an acute myocardial infarction has broad complex tachycardia it will almost always be ventricular tachycardia. However, a patient with episodes of broad complex tachycardia but without an infarction could have ventricular tachycardia, or supraventricular tachycardia with bundle branch block or the Wolff–Parkinson–White syndrome (see p. 79). Under such circumstances the following points may be helpful:

1. Finding P waves and seeing how they relate to the QRS complexes is always the key to identifying arrhythmias. Always look carefully at a full 12-lead ECG.
2. If possible, compare the QRS complex during the tachycardia with that during sinus rhythm. If the patient has bundle branch block when in sinus rhythm, the

QRS complex during the tachycardia will have the same shape as during normal rhythm.

3. If the QRS complex is wider than four small squares (160 ms), the rhythm will probably be ventricular in origin.
4. Left axis deviation during the tachycardia usually indicates a ventricular origin, as does any change of axis compared with a record taken during sinus rhythm.
5. If during the tachycardia the QRS complex is very irregular, the rhythm is probably atrial fibrillation with bundle branch block (see below).

FIBRILLATION

All the arrhythmias discussed so far have involved the synchronous contraction of all the muscle fibres of the atria or of the ventricles, albeit at abnormal speeds. When individual muscle fibres contract independently, they are said to be 'fibrillating'. Fibrillation can occur in the atrial or ventricular muscle.

ATRIAL FIBRILLATION

When the atrial muscle fibres contract independently there are no P waves on the ECG, only an irregular line (Fig. 3.25). At times there may be flutter-like waves for 2–3 s. The AV node is continuously bombarded with depolarization waves of varying strength, and depolarization spreads at irregular intervals down the His bundle. The AV node conducts in an 'all or none' fashion, so that the depolarization waves passing into the His bundle are of constant intensity. However, these waves are irregular, and the ventricles therefore contract irregularly. Because conduction into and through the ventricles is by the normal route, each QRS complex is of normal shape.

In a 12-lead record, fibrillation waves can often be seen much better in some leads than in others (Fig. 3.26).

Fig. 3.25

Atrial fibrillation

Lead II:

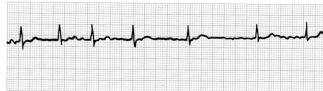

Lead V₁:

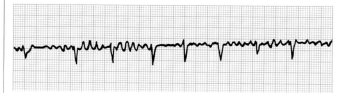

Note
- No P waves, and an irregular baseline
- Irregular QRS complexes
- Normally shaped QRS complexes
- In lead V₁, waves can be seen with some resemblance to those seen in atrial flutter – this is common in atrial fibrillation

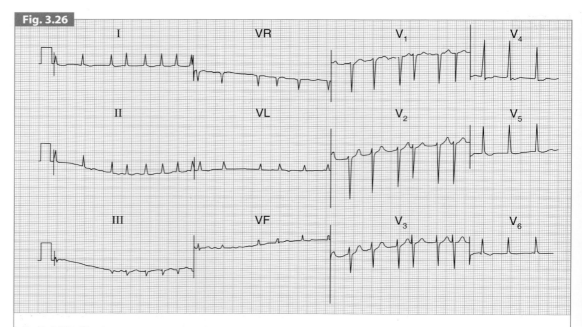

Fig. 3.26

Atrial fibrillation

Note

- No P waves
- Irregular baseline
- Irregular QRS complexes, rate varying between 75/min and 190/min
- Narrow QRS complexes of normal shape
- Depressed ST segments in leads V_5–V_6 (digoxin effect – see p. 101)
- Normal T waves

Fig. 3.27

Ventricular fibrillation

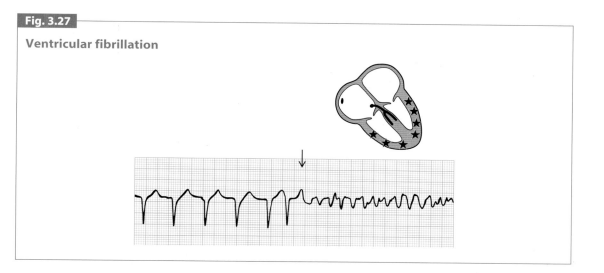

VENTRICULAR FIBRILLATION

When the ventricular muscle fibres contract independently, no QRS complex can be identified, and the ECG is totally disorganized (Fig. 3.27).

As the patient will usually have lost consciousness by the time you have realized that the change in the ECG pattern is not just due to a loose connection, the diagnosis is easy.

THE WOLFF–PARKINSON–WHITE (WPW) SYNDROME

The only normal electrical connection between the atria and ventricles is the His bundle. Some people, however, have an extra or 'accessory' conducting bundle, a condition known as the Wolff–Parkinson–White syndrome. The accessory bundles form a direct connection between the atrium and the ventricle, usually on the left side of the heart, and in these bundles there is no AV node to delay conduction. A depolarization wave therefore reaches the ventricle early, and 'pre-excitation' occurs. The PR interval is short, and the QRS complex shows an early slurred upstroke called a 'delta wave' (Fig. 3.28). The second part of the QRS complex is normal, as conduction through the His bundle catches up with the pre-excitation. The effects of the WPW syndrome on the ECG are considered in more detail in Chapter 7.

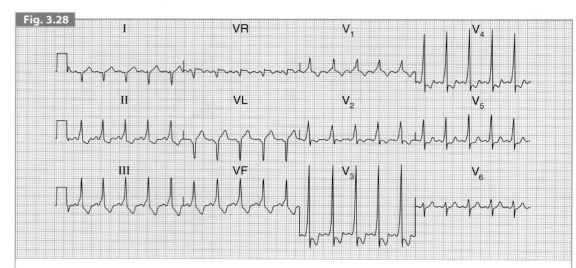

The Wolff–Parkinson–White syndrome

Note

- Sinus rhythm, rate 125/min
- Right axis deviation
- Short PR interval
- Slurred upstroke of the QRS complex, best seen in leads V_3 and V_4. Wide QRS complex due to this 'delta' wave
- Dominant R wave in lead V_1

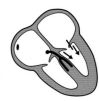

Fig. 3.29

Sustained tachycardia in the Wolff–Parkinson–White syndrome

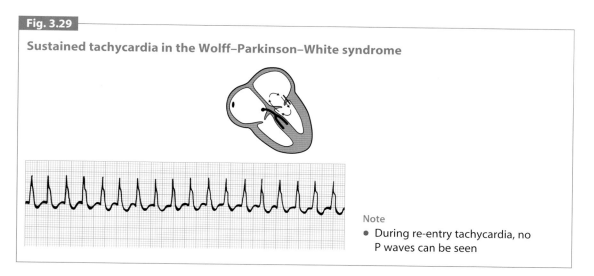

Note
- During re-entry tachycardia, no P waves can be seen

The only clinical importance of this anatomical abnormality is that it can cause paroxysmal tachycardia. Depolarization can spread down the His bundle and back up the accessory pathway, and so reactivate the atrium. A 're-entry' circuit is thus set up, and a sustained tachycardia occurs (Fig. 3.29).

THE ORIGINS OF TACHYCARDIAS

We have considered the tachycardias up to now as if all were due to an increased spontaneous frequency of depolarization of some part of the heart. While such an 'enhanced automaticity' certainly accounts for some tachycardias, others are due to re-entry circuits within the heart muscle. The tachycardias that we have described as 'junctional' are usually due to re-entry circuits around the AV node, and are therefore properly called 'atrioventricular nodal re-entry tachycardias' (AVNRTs). It is not possible to distinguish enhanced automaticity from re-entry tachycardia on standard ECGs, but fortunately this differentiation has no practical importance.

ECG
IP

For more on WPW syndrome, see pp. 69–72

WHAT TO DO

Accurate interpretation of the ECG is an essential part of arrhythmia management. Although this book is not intended to discuss therapy in detail, it seems appropriate to outline some simple approaches to patient management that logically follow interpretation of an ECG recording:

1. For fast or slow sinus rhythm, treat the underlying cause, not the rhythm itself.
2. Extrasystoles rarely need treatment.
3. In patients with acute heart failure or low blood pressure due to tachycardia, DC cardioversion should be considered early on.
4. Patients with any bradycardia that is affecting the circulation can be treated with atropine, but if this is ineffective they will need temporary or permanent pacing (Fig. 3.30).

5. The first treatment for any abnormal tachycardia is carotid sinus pressure. This should be performed with the ECG running, and may help make the diagnosis:
   - Sinus tachycardia: carotid sinus pressure causes temporary slowing of the heart rate.
   - Atrial and junctional tachycardia: carotid sinus pressure may terminate the arrhythmia or may have no effect.
   - Atrial flutter: carotid sinus pressure usually causes a temporary increase in block (e.g. from 2:1 to 3:1).
   - Atrial fibrillation and ventricular tachycardia: carotid sinus pressure has no effect.
6. Narrow complex tachycardias should be treated initially with adenosine.
7. Wide complex tachycardias should be treated initially with lidocaine.

ECG
IP

For more on pacemakers, see pp. 187–207

Fig. 3.30

Pacemaker

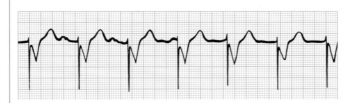

Note
- Occasional P waves are visible, but are not related to the QRS complexes
- The QRS complexes are preceded by a brief spike, representing the pacemaker stimulus
- The QRS complexes are broad, because pacemakers stimulate the right ventricle and cause 'ventricular' beats

REMINDERS

ABNORMAL CARDIAC RHYTHMS

- Most parts of the heart are capable of spontaneous depolarization.
- Abnormal rhythms can arise in the atrial muscle, the region around the AV node (the junctional region) and in the ventricular muscle.
- Escape rhythms are slow and are protective.
- Occasional early depolarization of any part of the heart causes an extrasystole.
- Frequent depolarization of any part of the heart causes tachycardia.
- Asynchronous contraction of muscle fibres in the atria or ventricles is called fibrillation.

- Apart from the rate, the ECG patterns of an escape rhythm, an extrasystole and a tachycardia arising in any one part of the heart are the same.
- All supraventricular rhythms have normal QRS complexes, provided there is no bundle branch block or pre-excitation (WPW) syndrome.
- Ventricular rhythms cause wide and abnormal QRS complexes, and abnormal T waves.

THE IDENTIFICATION OF RHYTHM ABNORMALITIES

Recognizing ECG abnormalities is to a large extent like recognizing an elephant – once seen, never forgotten. However, in cases of difficulty it is helpful to ask the following questions, referring to Table 3.1:

1. Is the abnormality occasional or sustained?
2. Are there any P waves?
3. Are there as many QRS complexes as P waves?
4. Are the ventricles contracting regularly or irregularly?
5. Is the QRS complex of normal shape?
6. What is the ventricular rate?

ECG
IP

For more on tachycardias, see pp. 113–147

Table 3.1 Recognizing ECG abnormalities

Abnormality	P wave	P:QRS ratio	QRS regularity	QRS shape	QRS rate	Rhythm
Occasional (i.e. extrasystoles)				Normal		Supraventricular
				Abnormal		Ventricular
Sustained	Present	P:QRS = 1:1	Regular	Normal	Normal	Sinus rhythm
					≥150/min	Atrial tachycardia
			Slightly irregular	Normal	Normal	Sinus arrhythmia
					Slow	Atrial escape
		More P waves than QRS complexes	Regular	Normal	Fast	Atrial tachycardia with block
					Slow	Second degree heart block
				Abnormal	Slow	Complete heart block
	Absent	n/a	Regular	Normal	Fast	Junctional tachycardia
					Slow	Junctional escape
				Abnormal	Fast	Junctional tachycardia with bundle branch block or ventricular tachycardia
			Irregular	Normal	Any speed	Atrial fibrillation
				Abnormal	Any speed	Atrial fibrillation and bundle branch block
		QRS complexes absent				Ventricular fibrillation or standstill

Abnormalities of P waves, QRS complexes and T waves

4

When interpreting an ECG, identify the rhythm first. Then ask the following questions – always in the same sequence:

1. Are there any abnormalities of the P wave?
2. What is the direction of the cardiac axis? (Look at the QRS complex in leads I, II and III – and at Ch. 1 if necessary.)
3. Is the QRS complex of normal duration?
4. Are there any abnormalities in the QRS complex – particularly, are there any abnormal Q waves?
5. Is the ST segment raised or depressed?
6. Is the T wave normal?

Remember:

1. The P wave can only be normal, unusually tall or unusually broad.
2. The QRS complex can only have three abnormalities – it can be too broad or too tall, and it may contain an abnormal Q wave.
3. The ST segment can only be normal, elevated or depressed.
4. The T wave can only be the right way up or the wrong way up.

ABNORMALITIES OF THE P WAVE

Apart from alterations of the shape of the P wave associated with rhythm changes, there are only two important abnormalities:

1. Anything that causes the right atrium to become hypertrophied (such as tricuspid valve stenosis or pulmonary hypertension) causes the P wave to become peaked (Fig. 4.1).
2. Left atrial hypertrophy (usually due to mitral stenosis) causes a broad and bifid P wave (Fig. 4.2).

Fig. 4.1

Right atrial hypertrophy

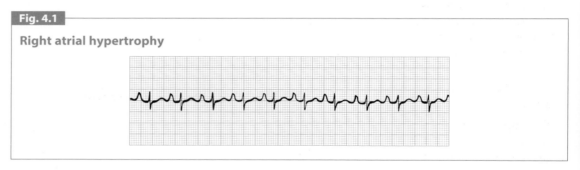

Fig. 4.2

Left atrial hypertrophy

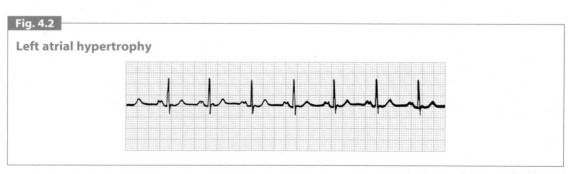

ABNORMALITIES OF THE QRS COMPLEX

The normal QRS complex has four characteristics:

1. Its duration is no greater than 120 ms (three small squares).
2. In a right ventricular lead (V_1), the S wave is greater than the R wave.
3. In a left ventricular lead (V_5 or V_6), the height of the R wave is less than 25 mm.
4. Left ventricular leads may show Q waves due to septal depolarization, but these are less than 1 mm across and less than 2 mm deep.

ABNORMALITIES OF THE WIDTH OF THE QRS COMPLEX

QRS complexes are abnormally wide in the presence of bundle branch block (see Ch. 2), or when depolarization is initiated by a focus in the ventricular muscle causing ventricular escape beats, extrasystoles or tachycardia (see Ch. 3). In each case, the increased width indicates that depolarization has spread through the ventricles by an abnormal and therefore slow pathway. The QRS complex is also wide in the Wolff–Parkinson–White syndrome (see p. 79, Ch. 3).

INCREASED HEIGHT OF THE QRS COMPLEX

An increase of muscle mass in either ventricle will lead to increased electrical activity, and to an increase in the height of the QRS complex.

Right ventricular hypertrophy

Right ventricular hypertrophy is best seen in the right ventricular leads (especially V_1). Since the left ventricle does not have its usual dominant effect on the QRS shape, the complex in lead V_1 becomes upright (i.e. the height of the R wave exceeds the depth of the S wave) – this is nearly always abnormal (Fig. 4.3). There will also be a deep S wave in lead V_6.

Fig. 4.3

The QRS complex in right ventricular hypertrophy

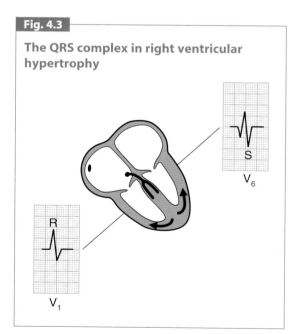

Right ventricular hypertrophy is usually accompanied by right axis deviation (see Ch. 1), by a peaked P wave (right atrial hypertrophy), and in severe cases by inversion of the T waves in leads V_1 and V_2, and sometimes in lead V_3 or even V_4 (Fig. 4.4).

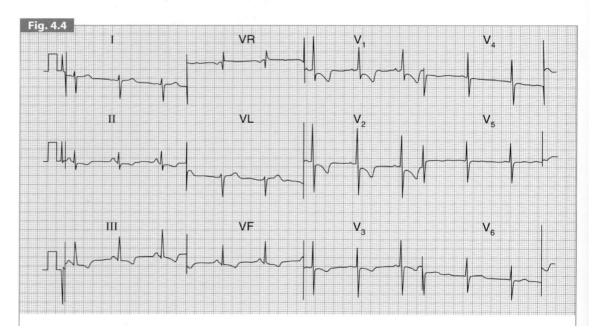

Fig. 4.4

Severe right ventricular hypertrophy

Note

- Sinus rhythm, rate 63/min
- Right axis deviation (deep S waves in lead I)
- Dominant R waves in lead V_1
- Deep S waves in lead V (clockwise rotation)
- Inverted T waves in leads II, III, VF and V_1–V_3
- Flat T waves in leads V_4–V_5

Pulmonary embolism

In pulmonary embolism the ECG may show features of right ventricular hypertrophy (Fig. 4.5), although in many cases there is nothing abnormal other than sinus tachycardia. When a pulmonary embolus is suspected, look for any of the following:

1. Peaked P waves.
2. Right axis deviation (S waves in lead I).
3. Tall R waves in lead V_1.
4. Right bundle branch block.
5. Inverted T waves in lead V_1 (normal), spreading across to lead V_2 or V_3.
6. A shift of transition point to the left, so that the R wave equals the S wave

Fig. 4.5

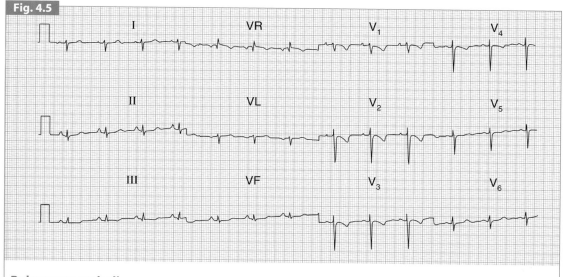

Pulmonary embolism

Note

- Sinus rhythm, rate 75/min
- Right axis deviation
- Peaked P waves, especially in lead II
- Persistent S wave in lead V_6
- T wave inversion in leads V_1–V_4

in lead V_5 or V_6 rather than in lead V_3 or V_4 (clockwise rotation). A deep S wave will persist in lead V_6.

7. Curiously, a 'Q' wave in lead III resembling an inferior infarction (see below).

However, do not hesitate to treat the patient if the clinical picture suggests pulmonary embolism but the ECG does not show the classical pattern of right ventricular hypertrophy. If in doubt, treat the patient with an anticoagulant.

Left ventricular hypertrophy

Left ventricular hypertrophy causes a tall R wave (greater than 25 mm) in lead V_5 or V_6 and a deep S wave in lead V_1 or V_2 (Fig. 4.6) – but in practice such 'voltage' changes alone are

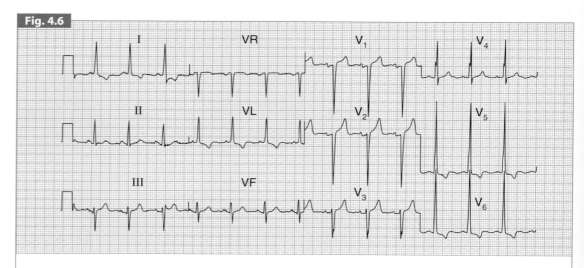

Fig. 4.6

Left ventricular hypertrophy

Note
- Sinus rhythm, rate 83/min
- Normal axis
- Tall R waves in leads V_5–V_6 (R wave in lead V_5, 40 mm) and deep S waves in leads V_1–V_2
- Inverted T waves in leads I, VL and V_5–V_6

unhelpful in diagnosing left ventricular enlargement. With significant hypertrophy, there are also inverted T waves in leads I, VL, V_5 and V_6, and sometimes V_4, and there may be left axis deviation. It is difficult to diagnose minor degrees of left ventricular hypertrophy from the ECG.

THE ORIGIN OF Q WAVES

Small (septal) 'Q' waves in the left ventricular leads result from depolarization of the septum from left to right (see Ch. 1). However, Q waves greater than one small square in width (representing 40 ms) and greater than 2 mm in depth have a quite different significance.

The ventricles are depolarized from inside outwards (Fig. 4.7). Therefore, an electrode placed in the cavity of a ventricle would record only a Q wave, because all the depolarization waves would be moving away from it. If a myocardial infarction causes complete death of muscle from the inside surface to the outside surface of the heart, an electrical 'window' is created, and an electrode looking at the heart over that window will record a cavity potential – that is, a Q wave.

Q waves greater than one small square in width and at least 2 mm deep therefore indicate a myocardial infarction, and the leads in which the Q wave appears give some indication of the part of the heart that has been damaged. Thus, infarction of the anterior wall of the left ventricle causes a Q wave in the leads looking

Fig. 4.7

The origin of Q waves

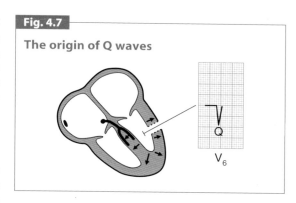

at the heart from the front – V_2–V_4 or V_5 (Fig. 4.8) (see Ch. 1).

If the infarction involves both the anterior and lateral surfaces of the heart, a Q wave will be present in leads V_3 and V_4 and in the leads that look at the lateral surface – I, VL and V_5–V_6 (Fig. 4.9).

Infarctions of the inferior surface of the heart cause Q waves in the leads looking at the heart from below – III and VF (Figs 4.8 and 4.10).

When the posterior wall of the left ventricle is infarcted, a different pattern is seen (Fig. 4.11). The right ventricle occupies the front of the heart anatomically, and normally depolarization of the right ventricle (moving towards the recording electrode V_1) is overshadowed by depolarization of the left ventricle (moving away from V_1). The result is a dominant S wave in lead V_1. With infarction of the posterior wall of the

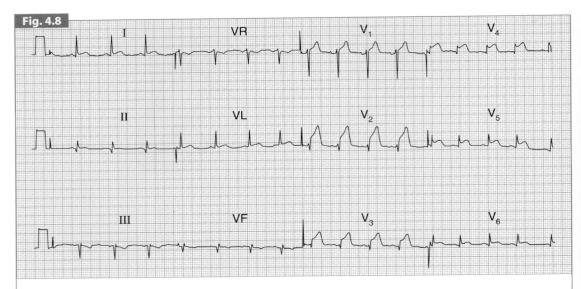

Fig. 4.8

Acute anterior myocardial infarction, and probable old inferior infarction

Note
- Sinus rhythm, rate 80/min
- Normal axis
- Small Q waves in leads II, III and VF – associated with flat ST segments and inverted T waves – indicate old inferior infarction
- Small Q waves in leads V_3–V_4 – associated with raised ST segments – indicate acute anterior infarction

ECG
IP

For more on myocardial infarction, see pp. 214–241

left ventricle, depolarization of the right ventricle is less opposed by left ventricular forces, and so becomes more obvious, and a dominant R wave develops in lead V_1. The appearance of the ECG is similar to that of right ventricular hypertrophy, though the other changes of right ventricular hypertrophy (see above) do not appear.

The presence of a Q wave does not give any indication of the age of an infarction, because once a Q wave has developed it is usually permanent.

Fig. 4.9

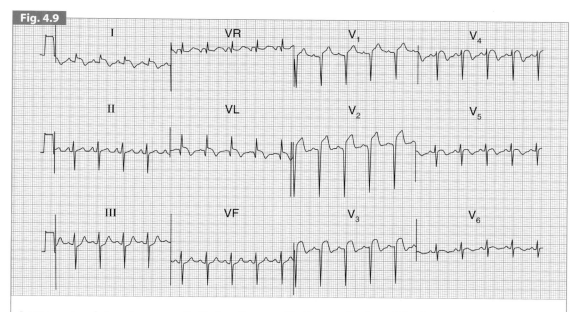

Acute anterolateral myocardial infarction and left anterior hemiblock

Note

- Sinus rhythm, rate 110/min
- Left axis deviation (dominant S waves in leads II and III)
- Q waves in leads VL and V_2–V_3
- Raised ST segments in leads I, VL and V_2–V_5

Fig. 4.10

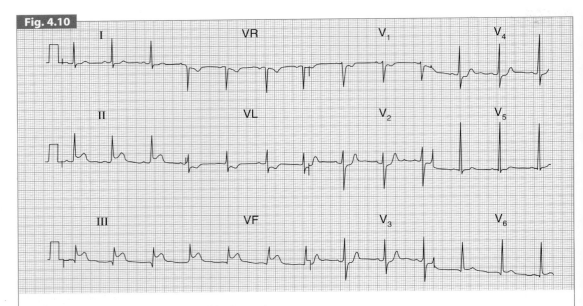

Acute inferior infarction; lateral ischaemia

Note

- Sinus rhythm, rate 70/min
- Normal axis
- Q waves in leads III and VF
- Normal QRS complexes
- Raised ST segments in leads II, III and VF
- Inverted T waves in lead VL (abnormal) and in lead V_1 (normal)

4

Fig. 4.11

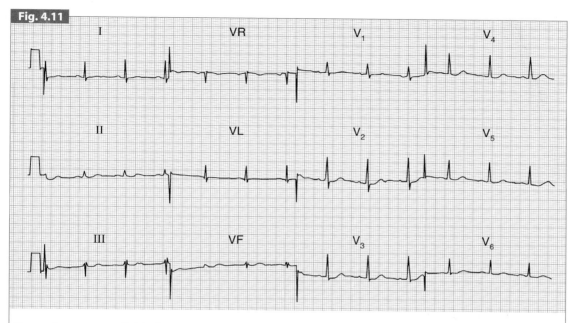

Posterior myocardial infarction

Note

- Sinus rhythm, rate 70/min
- Normal axis
- Dominant R waves in lead V_1
- Flattened T waves in leads I and VL

ABNORMALITIES OF THE ST SEGMENT

The ST segment lies between the QRS complex and the T wave (Fig. 4.12). It should be 'isoelectric' – that is, at the same level as the part between the T wave and the next P wave – but it may be elevated (Fig. 4.13a) or depressed (Fig. 4.13b).

Elevation of the ST segment is an indication of acute myocardial injury, usually due either to a recent infarction or to pericarditis. The leads in which the elevation occurs indicate the part

Fig. 4.12

The ST segment

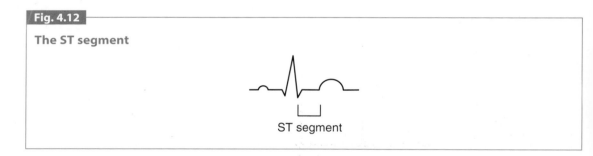

ST segment

Fig. 4.13

(a) Elevated ST segment. (b) Depressed ST segment

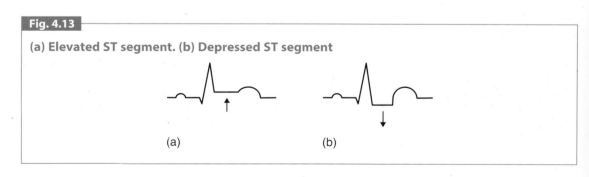

(a)   (b)

of the heart that is damaged – anterior damage shows in the V leads, and inferior damage in leads III and VF (see Figs 4.8 and 4.10). Pericarditis is not usually a localized affair, and so it causes ST elevation in most leads.

Horizontal depression of the ST segment, associated with an upright T wave, is usually a sign of ischaemia as opposed to infarction. When the ECG at rest is normal, ST segment depression may appear during exercise, particularly when effort induces angina (Fig. 4.14).

Downward-sloping – as opposed to horizontally depressed – ST segments are usually due to treatment with digoxin (see p. 101).

Fig. 4.14

Exercise-induced ischaemic changes

Rest:

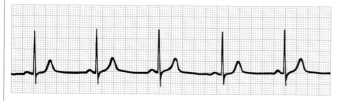

Exercise:

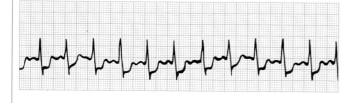

Note
- In the upper (normal) trace, the heart rate is 55/min and the ST segments are isoelectric
- In the lower trace, the heart rate is 125/min and the ST segments are horizontally depressed

ABNORMALITIES OF THE T WAVE

INVERSION OF THE T WAVE

The T wave is normally inverted in leads VR and V_1, sometimes in leads III and V_2, and also in lead V_3 in some black people.

T wave inversion is seen in the following circumstances:

1. Normality
2. Ischaemia
3. Ventricular hypertrophy
4. Bundle branch block
5. Digoxin treatment.

Leads adjacent to those showing inverted T waves sometimes show 'biphasic' T waves – initially upright and then inverted.

MYOCARDIAL INFARCTION

After a myocardial infarction, the first abnormality seen on the ECG is elevation of the ST segment (Fig. 4.15). Subsequently, Q waves appear, and the T waves become inverted. The ST segment returns to the baseline, the whole process taking a variable time but usually within the range 24–48 h. T wave inversion is often permanent. Infarctions causing this pattern of ECG changes are called 'ST segment elevation myocardial infarctions' (STEMIs) (see p. 130).

If an infarction is not full thickness and so does not cause an electrical window, there will be T wave inversion but no Q waves (Fig. 4.16). Infarctions with this pattern of ECG change are called 'non-ST segment elevation myocardial infarctions' (NSTEMIs). The older term for the same pattern was 'non-Q wave infarction' or 'subendocardial infarction'.

VENTRICULAR HYPERTROPHY

Left ventricular hypertrophy causes inverted T waves in leads looking at the left ventricle (I, II, VL, V_5–V_6) (see Fig. 4.6). Right ventricular hypertrophy causes T wave inversion in the leads looking at the right ventricle (T wave inversion is normal in lead V_1, and may be normal in lead V_2, but in white adults is abnormal in lead V_3) (see Fig. 4.4).

BUNDLE BRANCH BLOCK

The abnormal path of depolarization in bundle branch block is usually associated with an abnormal path of repolarization. Therefore, inverted T waves associated with QRS complexes which have a duration of 160 ms or more have no significance in themselves (see Figs 2.15 and 2.16).

Fig. 4.15

Development of inferior infarction

1 h after onset of pain:

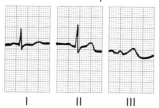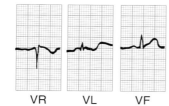

| I | II | III | VR | VL | VF |

6 h after onset of pain:

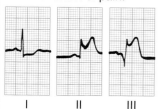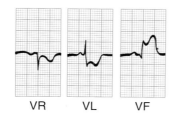

| I | II | III | VR | VL | VF |

24 h after onset of pain:

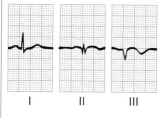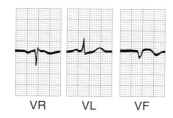

| I | II | III | VR | VL | VF |

Note

- Three ECGs have been recorded over 24 h, and have been arranged horizontally
- Sinus rhythm with a normal cardiac axis in all three ECGs
- The first record is essentially normal
- 6 h after the onset of pain, the ST segments have risen in leads II, III and VF, and the ST segment is depressed in leads I, VR and VL. A Q wave has developed in lead III
- 24 h after the onset of pain, a small Q wave has appeared in lead II, and more obvious Q waves can be seen in leads III and VF. The ST segments have returned to the baseline, and the T waves are now inverted in leads III and VF

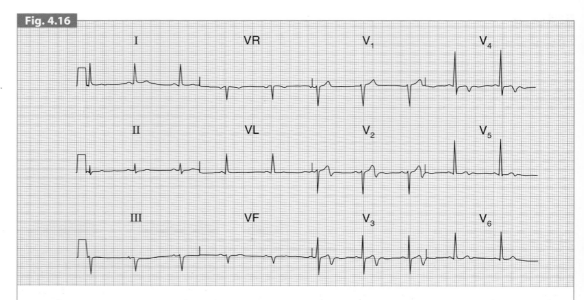

Fig. 4.16

Anterior non-ST segment elevation myocardial infarction

Note
- Sinus rhythm, rate 62/min
- Normal axis
- Normal QRS complexes
- Inverted T waves in leads V_3–V_4
- Biphasic T waves in leads V_2 and V_5

Fig. 4.17

Digoxin effect

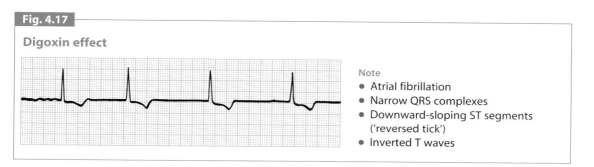

Note
- Atrial fibrillation
- Narrow QRS complexes
- Downward-sloping ST segments ('reversed tick')
- Inverted T waves

DIGOXIN

The administration of digoxin causes T wave inversion – characteristically with sloping depression of the ST segment (Fig. 4.17). It is helpful to record an ECG before giving digoxin, to save later confusion about the significance of T wave changes.

OTHER ABNORMALITIES OF THE ST SEGMENT AND THE T WAVE

ELECTROLYTE ABNORMALITIES

Abnormalities of the plasma levels of potassium, calcium and magnesium affect the ECG, though changes in the plasma sodium level do not. The T wave and QT interval (measured from the onset of the QRS complex to the end of the T wave) are most commonly affected.

A low potassium level causes T wave flattening and the appearance of a hump on the end of the T wave called a 'U' wave. A high potassium level causes peaked T waves with the disappearance of the ST segment. The QRS complex may be widened. The effects of abnormal magnesium levels are similar.

A low plasma calcium level causes prolongation of the QT interval, and a high plasma calcium level shortens it.

NONSPECIFIC CHANGES

Minor degrees of ST segment and T wave abnormalities (T wave flattening, etc.) are usually of no great significance, and are best reported as 'nonspecific ST–T changes'.

101

REMINDERS

CAUSES OF ABNORMAL P WAVES, QRS COMPLEXES AND T WAVES

- Tall P waves result from right atrial hypertrophy, and broad P waves from left atrial hypertrophy.
- Broadening of the QRS complex indicates abnormal intraventricular conduction: it is seen in bundle branch block and in complexes originating in the ventricular muscle. It is also seen in the Wolff–Parkinson–White syndrome.
- Increased height of the QRS complex indicates ventricular hypertrophy. Right ventricular hypertrophy is seen in lead V_1, and left ventricular hypertrophy is seen in leads V_5–V_6.
- Q waves greater than 1 mm across and 2 mm deep indicate myocardial infarction.
- ST segment elevation indicates acute myocardial infarction or pericarditis.

- ST segment depression and T wave inversion may be due to ischaemia, ventricular hypertrophy, abnormal intraventricular conduction, or digoxin.
- T wave inversion is normal in leads III, VR and V_1. T wave inversion is associated with bundle branch block, ischaemia, and ventricular hypertrophy.
- T wave flattening or peaking with an unusually long or short QT interval may be due to electrolyte abnormalities, but many minor ST–T changes are nonspecific.

AND REMEMBER

- The ECG is easy to understand.
- Most abnormalities of the ECG are amenable to reason.

ECG
IP

For more on the effect of electrolyte abnormalities, see pp. 331–334

Making the most of the ECG

The clinical interpretation of individual ECGs

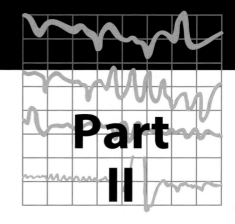

Part II

In practical terms the ECG is simply a tool for the diagnosis and treatment of patients, and must always be considered in the light of the patient's history and the physical findings. This is because identical ECG appearances – 'normal' or otherwise – can be seen in healthy and in ill patients.

In this part of the book, we look beyond the basics and consider how the ECG can help in the situations in which it is most used – in the 'screening' of healthy subjects, and in patients with chest pain, breathlessness, palpitations or syncope. Recalling the classic ECG abnormalities covered in Part I, we will look at some of the variations that can make ECG interpretation seem more difficult, using examples of more ECGs from patients with common problems.

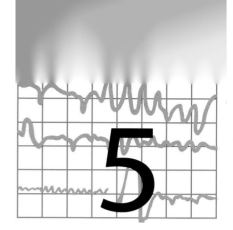

The ECG in healthy subjects

The ECG is frequently used in 'health screening', but it is important to remember that not all those who are screened are really asymptomatic – the procedure may be used as an alternative to seeking medical advice. On the other hand, people being screened may be totally free of symptoms and yet important abnormalities may be evident from their ECGs. For example, Figure 5.1 shows the ECG of an asymptomatic patient which, quite unexpectedly, revealed atrial fibrillation. Abnormalities are uncommon in this group of individuals, but perhaps are the best reason for using the ECG in screening. All the ECGs in this chapter came from health screening clinics, and we will assume that the individuals considered themselves to be healthy.

THE NORMAL CARDIAC RHYTHM

Sinus rhythm is the only truly normal rhythm. 'Sinus bradycardia' is sometimes said to be present when the heart rate is below 60/min, and 'sinus tachycardia' is sometimes used for heart rates above 100/min (Box 5.1), but these terms are really not helpful, and it is far more useful to describe a patient as having 'sinus rhythm at x/min' (Fig. 5.2).

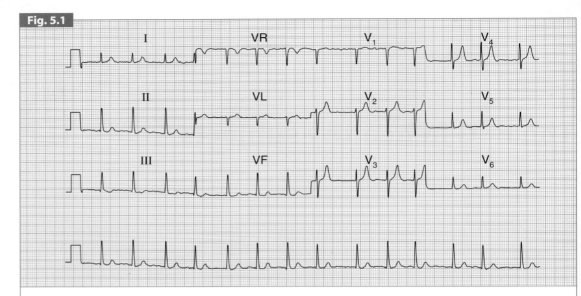

Fig. 5.1

Atrial fibrillation in an asymptomatic subject

Note

- Atrial fibrillation
- Ventricular rate about 85/min
- Normal QRS complexes and T waves
- There is no ST segment depression, suggesting that the individual is not taking digoxin

Fig. 5.2

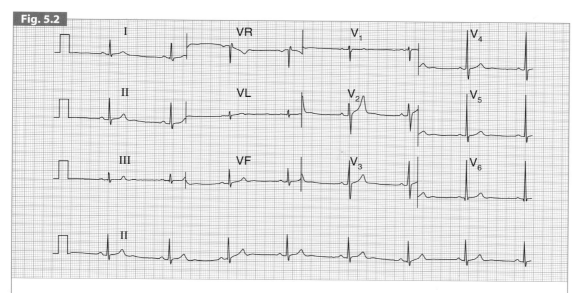

Sinus bradycardia in an athlete

Note
- Sinus rhythm, rate 47/min
- Normal QRS complexes, ST segments and T waves

Box 5.1 Causes of sinus bradycardia or tachycardia

Sinus bradycardia	Sinus tachycardia
• Physical fitness	• Exercise, pain, fright
• Vasovagal attacks	• Obesity
• Hypothermia	• Pregnancy
• Hypothyroidism	• Anaemia
	• Thyrotoxicosis
	• CO_2 retention

EXTRASYSTOLES

Supraventricular extrasystoles are of no clinical significance, although atrial extrasystoles need to be differentiated from the variations in beat-to-beat interval which occur in sinus rhythm (Figs 5.3 and 5.4). Automated ECG reporting often fails to do this.

Occasional ventricular extrasystoles are experienced by many people with normal hearts. Frequent ventricular extrasystoles (Fig. 5.5) may indicate heart disease, and in a large population

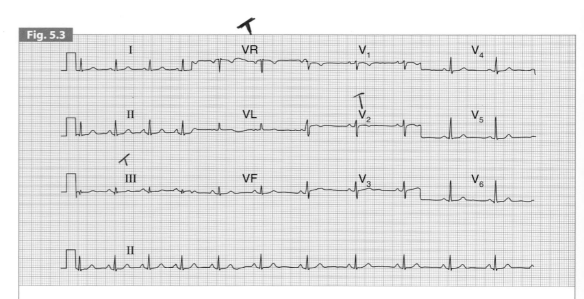

Fig. 5.3

Sinus arrhythmia

Note
- Sinus rhythm, rate about 65/min overall
- The lead II rhythm strip shows that the rate is initially about 80/min but slows progressively to 60/min
- The QRS complexes, ST segments and T waves are normal

their presence does identify a group with a higher than average risk of developing cardiac problems. In an individual patient, however, their presence is not a good predictor of such risk.

Extrasystoles may disappear if alcohol or coffee intake is reduced, and only need treating medically when they are so frequent as to impair cardiac function.

Fig. 5.4

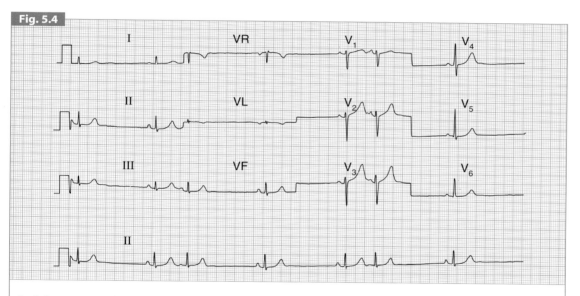

Atrial extrasystoles
Note
- Sinus rhythm; rate as judged from adjacent sinus beats is about 35/min
- The overall heart rate, calculated including the extrasystoles, is about 45/min
- Extrasystoles are identified by early P waves that are differently shaped compared with those associated with the sinus beats
- The QRS complexes and T waves are the same in the sinus and atrial beats

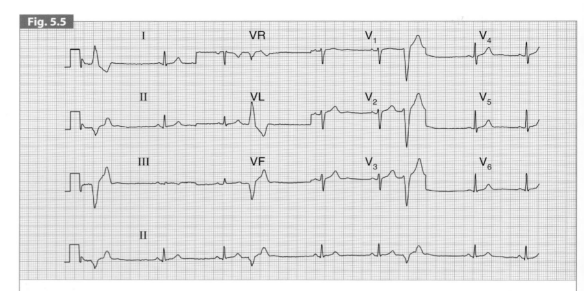

Fig. 5.5

Ventricular extrasystoles

Note

- Sinus rhythm, rate 50/min
- Frequent ventricular extrasystoles, identified by their early occurrence without preceding P waves, and by their wide and abnormal QRS complex and differently shaped T wave compared with the sinus beats
- In the sinus beats the QRS complexes and T waves are normal

ECTOPIC ATRIAL RHYTHM

When depolarization is initiated from a focus in the atrium rather than in the sinoatrial node, an 'ectopic atrial rhythm' is present (Fig. 5.6). This does not cause symptoms and is usually of no clinical significance. It is not an uncommon finding in individuals being screened.

Fig. 5.6

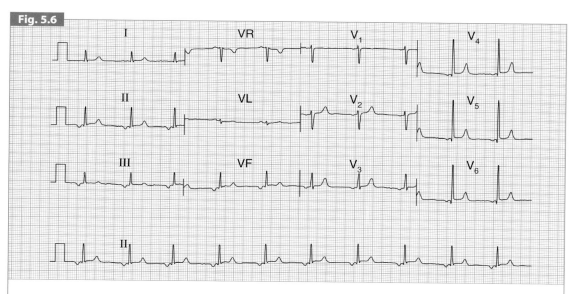

Ectopic atrial rhythm

Note
- Regular rhythm with inverted P waves in most leads, indicating that an atrial focus controls the heart rate
- The PR interval is at the lower end of normal, at 140 ms
- Heart rate 60/min
- The QRS complexes, ST segments and T waves are all normal

THE P WAVE

Tall P waves may be due to right atrial hypertrophy, and are significant if there is evidence of right ventricular hypertrophy as well. Tall P waves alone may indicate tricuspid stenosis, but this is rare. If the patient is well and has no abnormal physical signs, 'tall' P waves are probably within the normal limits.

Bifid P waves in the absence of signs of associated left ventricular hypertrophy can indicate mitral stenosis (now fairly rare), but a bifid and not particularly prolonged P wave is often seen in the anterior leads of normal ECGs. Figure 5.7 shows the ECG of an asymptomatic patient with a clinically normal heart.

The P waves of atrial extrasystoles tend to be abnormally shaped compared to the P waves of the sinus beats of the same patient (Fig. 5.4).

P waves cannot always be seen in all leads, but if there is a total absence of P waves the rhythm is probably not sinus and may be sinus arrest, junctional escape or atrial fibrillation; or the patient may have hyperkalaemia.

CONDUCTION

The upper limit of the PR interval in a normal ECG is usually taken as 220 ms, a longer PR interval indicating first degree heart block. However, the ECGs of healthy individuals, especially athletes, not uncommonly have PR intervals slightly longer than 220 ms, and these can be ignored in the absence of any other indication of heart disease.

The ECG in Figure 5.8 was recorded from a healthy, asymptomatic individual at a screening examination. Nevertheless, PR interval prolongation to this extent is probably evidence of disease of the conducting tissue.

Second degree heart block of the Mobitz 1 (Wenckebach) type may be seen in athletes, but otherwise second and third degree block are indications of heart disease.

For an example mitral stenosis, see p. 293

For more on hyperkalaemia, see p. 331

Fig. 5.7

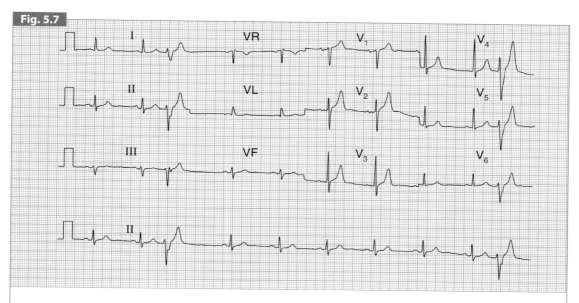

Bifid P waves

Note

- Sinus rhythm, rate 60/min
- There are two ventricular extrasystoles
- In leads V_2, V_3 and V_4 the P wave is 'bifid'. This can be a sign of left atrial hypertrophy, but is often seen in normal ECGs
- In the sinus beats the QRS complexes, ST segments and T waves are normal

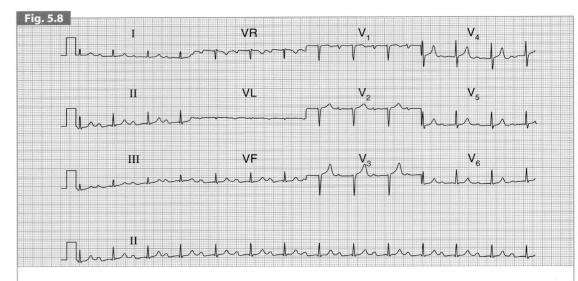

Fig. 5.8

First degree heart block

Note
- Sinus rhythm, rate 80/min
- PR interval prolonged at 336 ms
- Constant PR interval in all beats
- Loss of the R wave in lead V_3 could indicate an old anterior infarction, otherwise QRS complexes, ST segments and T waves are normal

A QRS complex that is predominantly downward (that is, the S wave is greater than the R wave) in leads II and III indicates left axis deviation, and a downward QRS complex in lead II, still within the normal limit of 120 ms, indicates left anterior hemiblock (Fig. 5.9).

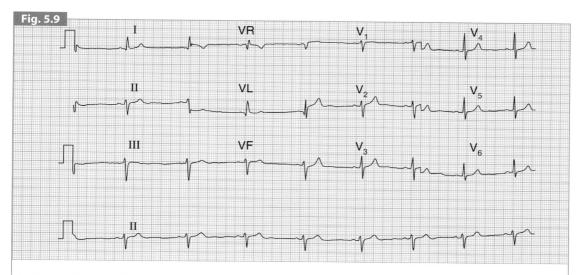

Fig. 5.9

Left anterior hemiblock

Note
- Sinus rhythm, rate 50/min
- QRS complexes upright in lead I, but mainly downward in leads II and III, indicating left axis deviation
- Slightly wide QRS complexes (but still within the normal limit of 120 ms) indicate left anterior hemiblock
- QRS complexes and T waves are otherwise normal

Right axis deviation is indicated if the QRS complexes are predominantly downward in lead I. It is common in healthy subjects, particularly if they are tall, as with the ECG in Figure 5.10, and under these circumstances is unimportant unless there is some other evidence of right ventricular hypertrophy, or the patient has had a myocardial infarction, raising the possibility of left posterior hemiblock.

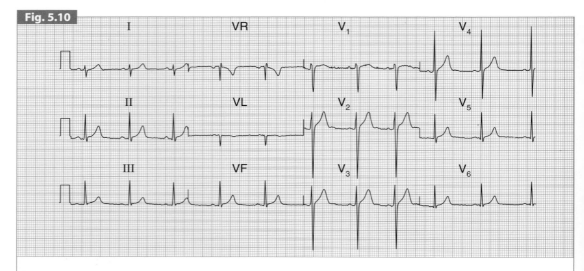

Fig. 5.10

Right axis deviation

Note

- Sinus rhythm, rate 60/min
- QRS complexes predominantly downward (S wave greater than R wave) in lead I

- Upright QRS complexes (R wave greater than S wave) in leads II–III
- QRS complexes and T waves are normal

THE QRS COMPLEX

Depolarization of the whole ventricular muscle mass should occur within 120 ms, so this represents the maximum width of the normal QRS complex. Any widening indicates conduction delay or failure within the bundle branch system, pre-excitation (see below), or a ventricular origin of depolarization – any of which may be seen in healthy subjects.

Left bundle branch block is always a sign of heart disease. Right bundle branch block with a QRS complex duration greater than 120 ms is sometimes seen in healthy subjects, but should be taken as a warning of things like an atrial septal defect. Partial (incomplete) right bundle branch block (RSR[1] pattern in lead V_1, but with a QRS complex duration less than 120 ms; Fig. 5.11) is very common and of no significance (Box 5.2).

Fig. 5.11

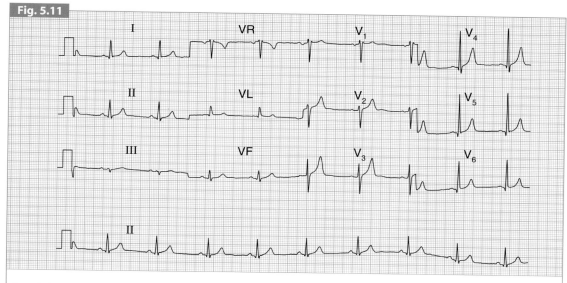

Partial right bundle branch block

Note

- Sinus rhythm, rate 55/min
- Normal cardiac axis
- RSR[1] pattern in lead V_1, but the QRS complex duration is normal at 100 ms
- QRS complexes, ST segments and T waves are otherwise normal

Box 5.2 **Causes of bundle branch block**

Right bundle branch block	**Left bundle branch block**
• Normal heart	• Ischaemia
• Atrial septal defect and other congenital disease	• Aortic stenosis
• Pulmonary embolism	• Hypertension
	• Cardiomyopathy

The height of the QRS complex is related to the thickness of heart muscle, but is actually a poor indicator of ventricular hypertrophy.

Right ventricular hypertrophy causes a dominant R wave in lead V_1, but unless there are other significant ECG signs (right axis deviation, or T wave inversion in leads V_2–V_3), this can be a normal variant (Fig. 5.12).

One ECG feature of left ventricular hypertrophy is the increased height of the QRS complex in the leads that 'look at' the left ventricle (Fig. 5.13), the generally accepted upper limit of normality being a QRS complex height of 25 mm in lead V_5 or V_6. The Sokolow–Lyon criteria define left ventricular hypertrophy as being present when the sum of

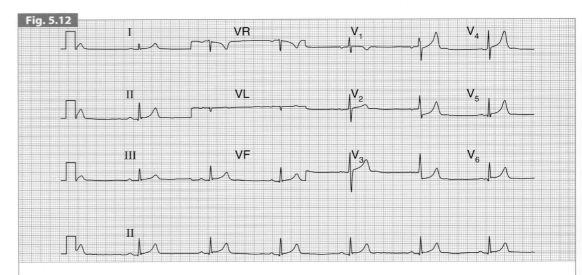

Fig. 5.12

Normal ECG with dominant R wave in lead V_1

Note
- Sinus rhythm, rate 40/min
- Normal cardiac axis (QRS complexes upright in leads I–III)
- Dominant (i.e. predominantly upright) R wave in lead V_1
- QRS complexes, ST segments and T waves otherwise normal – no other evidence of right ventricular hypertrophy

the R wave height in lead V_5 or V_6 plus the depth of the S wave in lead V_1 exceeds 35 mm. In fact these criteria are unreliable, and a QRS complex height greater than 25 mm is often seen in fit young men. Left ventricular hypertrophy can only be diagnosed with confidence when tall QRS complexes are associated with inverted T waves in the lateral leads (see Ch. 4). This is sometimes referred to as a 'strain' pattern, but this term is essentially meaningless.

If the QRS complexes seem too small to be consistent with the clinical findings, check the calibration of the ECG recorder. If this is correct, possible explanations of small QRS complexes are obesity, emphysema and pericardial effusion.

Q waves are the hallmark of the fully developed changes of an ST segment elevation

ECG
IP

For more on left ventricular hypertrophy, see pp. 295–302

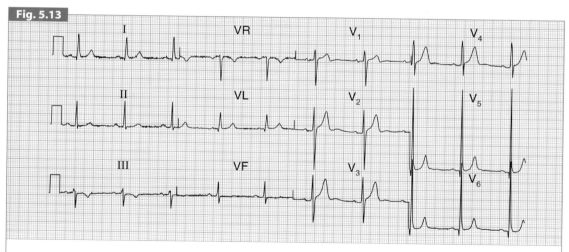

Fig. 5.13

Normal ECG with increased height of QRS complexes

Note
- Sinus rhythm, rate 60/min
- Normal cardiac axis
- QRS complex: R wave in lead V_5 = 45 mm; S wave in lead V_1 = 15 mm. This is left ventricular hypertrophy on voltage criteria, but there is no T wave inversion to suggest significant left ventricular hypertrophy

myocardial infarction, but they also result from septal depolarization (see p. 17). Narrow Q waves in the inferior and lateral leads (Fig. 5.14), and sometimes even quite deep ones, may also be perfectly normal.

A Q wave in lead III but not in lead VF is likely to be normal, even when associated with an inverted T wave (Fig. 5.15). These features often disappear if the ECG is repeated with the subject taking and holding in a deep breath.

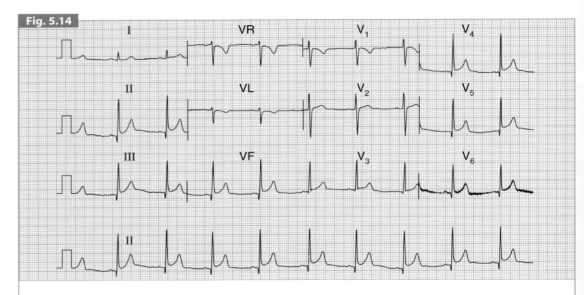

Fig. 5.14

Normal ECG with marked infero-lateral Q waves

Note
- Sinus rhythm, rate 60/min
- Normal cardiac axis
- QRS complexes in leads II, III, VF and V_4–V_6 show deep but narrow Q waves
- Normal ST segments and T waves
- Lead V_6 shows electrical interference

Fig. 5.15

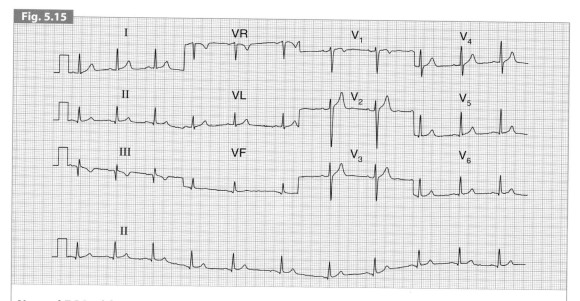

Normal ECG with Q wave and inverted T wave in lead III

Note

- Sinus rhythm, rate 65/min
- The QRS complex in lead III shows a Q wave, and lead VF has a very small Q wave. Otherwise the QRS complexes are normal
- There are inverted T waves in leads III, VR and V$_1$, but not elsewhere

THE ST SEGMENT

If the ST segment is raised following an S wave it is described as 'high take-off', and is a normal variant (Fig. 5.16); this pattern is typically seen in the anterior leads. It is important to differentiate this from the raised ST segment of an ST segment elevation myocardial infarction.

Horizontal ST segment depression is a sign of ischaemia (see Ch. 4), but minor degrees of depression, often downward-sloping, are seen in the ECGs of normal people, and are best described as 'nonspecific' (Fig. 5.17).

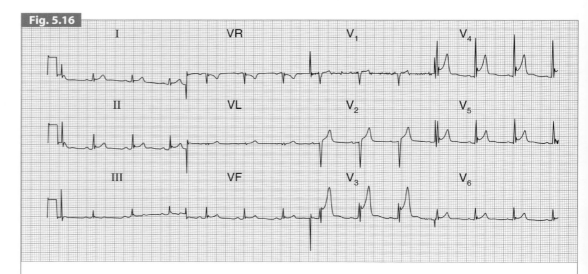

Fig. 5.16

Normal ECG with high take-off ST segments

Note

- Sinus rhythm, rate 75/min
- Normal axis
- Normal QRS complexes
- In leads V_3–V_5 there is a small S wave followed by a small secondary R wave
- The ST segment begins 5 mm above the baseline in lead V_3, and 2 mm above the baseline in leads V_4–V_5

Fig. 5.17

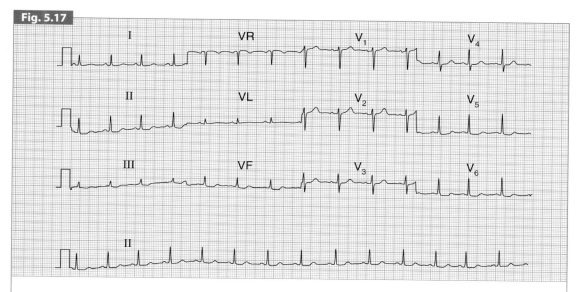

Normal ECG with nonspecific ST segment changes

Note

- Sinus rhythm, rate 85/min
- Normal axis
- Normal QRS complexes
- In leads II, III, VF and V_5–V_6 there is slight downward-sloping ST segment depression
- Normal T waves

THE T WAVE

The T wave is almost always inverted in lead VR, usually in lead V_1 and sometimes in lead III. Occasionally, a normal heart may be associated with an inverted T wave in lead V_2, and in black people there may be T wave inversion in leads V_3 and V_4 as well (Fig. 5.18). This can lead to an incorrect diagnosis of a non-ST segment elevation myocardial infarction (non-Q wave infarction).

Tall and peaked T waves (Fig. 5.19) are sometimes seen in the early stages of a myocardial infarction, when they may be

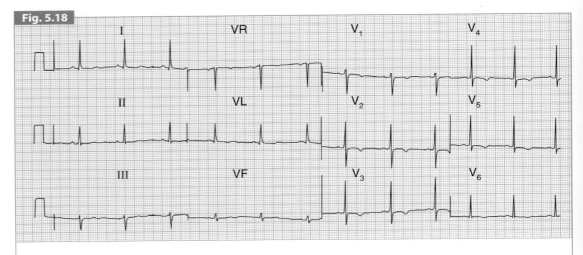

Fig. 5.18

Normal ECG from a black man

Note
- Sinus rhythm, rate 62/min
- Normal axis (there is a dominant S wave in lead III, but a dominant R wave in lead II)
- Normal QRS complexes and ST segments
- T wave inversion in all the chest leads, especially V_2–V_5
- In a white man this might suggest a non-ST segment elevation myocardial infarction, but in a black man it is perfectly normal

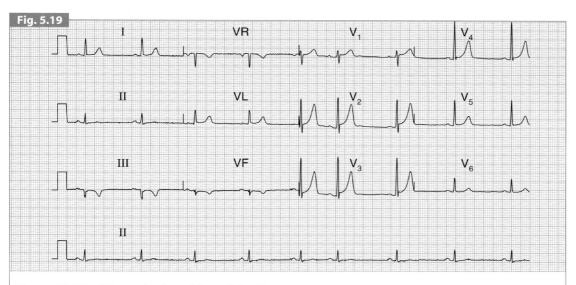

Fig. 5.19

Normal ECG with marked peaking of the T waves

Note

- Sinus rhythm, rate 50/min, with one atrial extrasystole
- Normal axis (QRS complexes predominantly downward in lead III, but upright in leads I and II)

- Normal QRS complexes
- High take-off ST segments in leads V_1–V_4
- Peaked T waves in leads V_2–V_4

described as 'hyperacute' changes. Peaked T waves are also associated with hyperkalaemia, but in fact some of the tallest and most peaked T waves are seen in perfectly normal ECGs.

U WAVES

Flat U waves following flat T waves, together with a prolonged QT interval, may be a sign of hypokalaemia. However, the best examples of prominent U waves come from normal people (Fig. 5.20).

THE ECG IN ATHLETES

Athletes' ECGs can show a wide variety of changes that could be considered 'abnormal' (see Box 5.3).

For more on hypokalaemia, see pp. 331–334

125

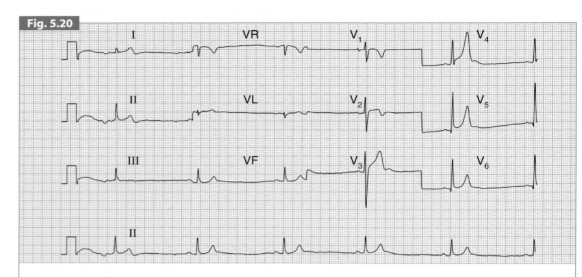

Fig. 5.20

Normal ECG with prominent U waves

Note

- The ECG appearance at the beginning is due to movement of the patient
- Sinus rhythm, rate 35/min (sinus bradycardia)
- Normal axis

- Normal QRS complexes
- Peaked T waves in leads V_4–V_6
- Prominent U waves in leads V_3–V_5

Box 5.3 Possible ECG features of healthy athletes

Variations in rhythm	Other variations in the ECG
• Sinus bradycardia	• Tall P waves and QRS complexes
• Junctional rhythm	• Prominent septal Q waves
• 'Wandering' atrial pacemaker	• Counterclockwise rotation
• First degree block	• Tall symmetrical T waves
• Mobitz type 1 (Wenckebach) second degree block	• Biphasic T waves
	• T wave inversion in the lateral leads
	• Prominent U waves

REMINDERS
THE NORMAL ECG

Limits of normal durations
- PR interval: 220 ms.
- QRS complex duration: 120 ms.
- QT_c interval: 450 ms.

Rhythm
- Sinus arrhythmia.
- Supraventricular extrasystoles are always normal.

The cardiac axis
- Normal axis: QRS complexes predominantly upward in leads I, II and III; still normal if the QRS complex is downward in lead III.
- Minor degrees of right and left axis deviation are within the normal range.

QRS complex
- Small Q waves are normal in leads I, VL and V_6 (septal Q waves).
- RSR^1 pattern in lead V_1 is normal if the duration is less than 120 ms (partial right bundle branch block).
- R wave is smaller than S wave in lead V_1.
- R wave in lead V_6 is less than 25 mm.
- R wave in lead V_6 plus S wave in lead V_1 is less than 35 mm.

ST segment
- Should be isoelectric.

T wave
- May be inverted in:
  - lead III
  - lead VR
  - lead V_1
  - leads V_2 and V_3, in black people.

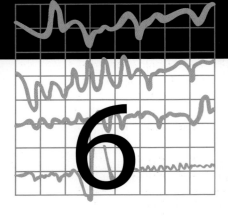

6

The ECG in patients with chest pain or breathlessness

Chest pain is a very common complaint, and when reviewing the ECG of a patient with chest pain it is essential to remember that there are causes other than myocardial ischaemia (Box 6.1).

There are a few features of chest pain that make the diagnosis obvious. Chest pain that radiates to the teeth or jaw is probably cardiac in origin; pain that is worse on inspiration is either pleuritic or due to pericarditis; and pain in the back may be due to either myocardial ischaemia or aortic dissection. The ECG will help to differentiate these causes of pain but it is not infallible – for example, if an aortic

Box 6.1 **Causes of chest pain**

Acute chest pain	**Intermittent chest pain**
• Myocardial infarction	• Angina
• Pulmonary embolism	• Oesophageal pain
• Pneumothorax and other pleuritic disease	• Muscular pain
• Pericarditis	• Nonspecific pain
• Aortic dissection	

dissection affects the coronary artery ostia, it can cause myocardial ischaemia.

THE ECG IN PATIENTS WITH CONSTANT CHEST PAIN

THE ECG IN ACUTE CORONARY SYNDROMES

'Acute coronary syndrome' is a term that covers a spectrum of clinical conditions caused by the rupture of atheromatous plaque within a coronary artery. On the exposed core of the plaque, a thrombus forms, and this can cause total or partial occlusion of the artery. The clinical syndrome ranges from angina at rest (unstable angina) to transmural myocardial infarction, and some definitions of acute coronary syndrome also include sudden death due to coronary occlusion. The diagnosis of acute coronary syndrome is based on the clinical presentation (including a previous history of coronary disease), ECG changes, and biochemical markers, principally troponin.

If a patient has chest pain and there is ECG evidence of myocardial ischaemia but a normal plasma troponin level, then the diagnosis is acute coronary syndrome due to unstable angina. Myocardial necrosis causes a rise in the level of plasma troponin (either troponin T or troponin I), and a high-sensitivity assay can detect a very small rise. By some definitions, any such rise in a clinical situation suggesting myocardial ischaemia justifies a diagnosis of myocardial infarction. However, the plasma troponin level may also rise in other conditions, which may also be associated with chest pain (Box 6.2). It is essential to remember that the plasma troponin level may not rise for up to 12 h after the onset of chest pain due to a myocardial infarction.

Thus the ECG is an essential tool in the diagnosis of an acute coronary syndrome. Importantly, it also distinguishes between two categories of myocardial infarction whose management is different. The first is infarction associated with ST segment elevation, known as 'ST segment elevation myocardial infarction' or 'STEMI', and the second is 'non-ST segment elevation myocardial infarction' or 'NSTEMI'. Differentiation is important because a STEMI requires immediate treatment by thrombolysis or percutaneous intervention (PCI – i.e. angioplasty and probably stenting), although after 6 h the benefit of this treatment is largely lost. An NSTEMI may also require PCI but with

Box 6.2 Common causes of plasma troponin level elevation in the absence of acute myocardial infarction

- Acute pulmonary embolism
- Acute pericarditis
- Acute or severe heart failure
- Sepsis and/or shock
- Renal failure
- False positive (laboratory problems, including the presence of heterophilic antibodies and rheumatoid factor)

considerably less urgency, and the patient is initially treated with some form of heparin, anti-platelet agents and a beta-blocker.

During the first few hours after the onset of chest pain due to myocardial infarction the ECG can remain apparently normal, and for this reason ECGs should be recorded repeatedly in a patient with chest pain that could be due to cardiac ischaemia, but whose ECG is nondiagnostic.

UNSTABLE ANGINA

In unstable angina there is ST segment depression while the patient has pain (Fig. 6.1). Once the pain has resolved the ECG returns to normal, or to its previous state if the patient has had a myocardial infarction in the past.

STEMI

In STEMI the ST segments rise in the ECG leads corresponding to the part of the heart that is damaged: the V leads with anterior infarction, lead VL and the lateral chest leads with lateral infarction, and leads III and VF with inferior infarction. STEMI is diagnosed when there is more than 1 mm of ST segment elevation in at least two contiguous limb leads (e.g. I and VL; III and VF), or more than 2 mm of ST segment elevation in at least two contiguous precordial leads. The diagnosis of STEMI can also be accepted if there is left bundle branch block which is known to be new.

Prompt treatment by PCI or thrombolysis may prevent myocardial damage, so that Q waves do not develop. Otherwise, after a variable time, usually within a day or so, the ST segments return to the baseline, the T waves in the affected leads become inverted, and Q waves develop (see p. 91). Once Q waves and inverted T waves have developed following infarction, these ECG changes are usually permanent. If anterior ST segment elevation persists, a left ventricular aneurysm should be suspected.

Figures 6.2–6.5 show ECGs from different patients with anterior infarctions, at increasing times from the onset of symptoms.

An old anterior infarction can also be diagnosed from an ECG that shows a loss of R wave development in the anterior leads without the presence of Q waves (Fig. 6.6). These changes must be differentiated from those due to chronic lung disease, in which the characteristic change is a persistent S wave in lead V_6. This is sometimes called 'clockwise rotation' because the heart has rotated so that the right ventricle occupies more of the precordium, and seen from below the rotation is clockwise (Fig. 6.7).

Fig. 6.1

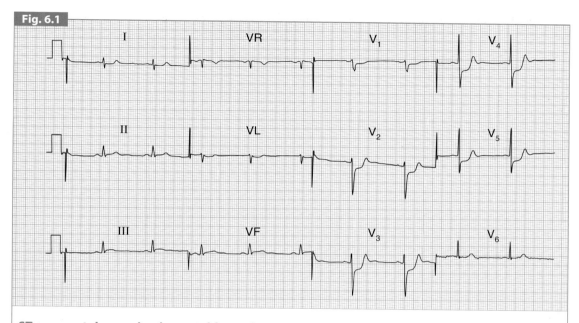

ST segment depression in unstable angina

Note

- Sinus rhythm, rate 60/min
- Normal axis
- Normal QRS complexes
- ST segments depressed horizontally in leads V_3–V_5
- Normal T waves

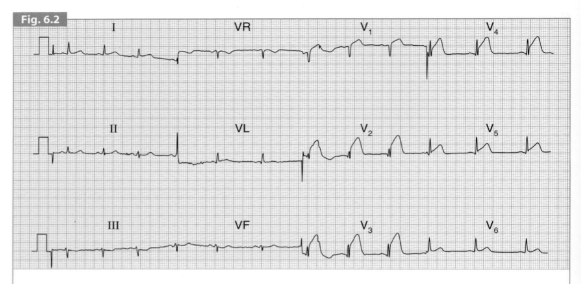

ST segment elevation in acute anterior ST segment elevation myocardial infarction

Note

- Sinus rhythm, rate 75/min
- Normal axis
- Normal QRS complexes
- ST segments elevated in leads V_1–V_5
- Normal T waves
- The ST segment elevation could be confused with high take-off ST segments, but the trace has to be interpreted in the context of a patient with acute chest pain

Fig. 6.3

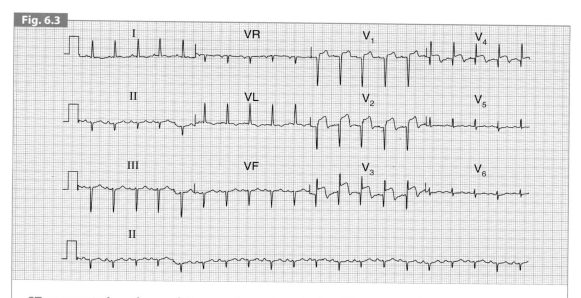

ST segment elevation and Q waves in acute anterior ST segment elevation myocardial infarction

Note

- Sinus rhythm, rate 120/min
- Left axis deviation (predominantly downward deflection in leads II and III)
- Q waves in leads V_1–V_4
- Raised ST segments in leads V_2–V_4
- Inverted T wave in lead VL, and biphasic T wave in lead V_3

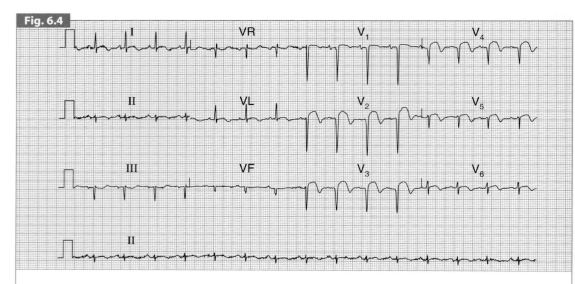

Fig. 6.4

ST segment elevation and marked Q waves in acute anterior ST segment elevation myocardial infarction

Note

- Sinus rhythm, rate 90/min
- Normal axis
- Deep Q waves and loss of R waves in leads V_1–V_4
- Raised ST segments in leads I, VL and V_2–V_6

Fig. 6.5

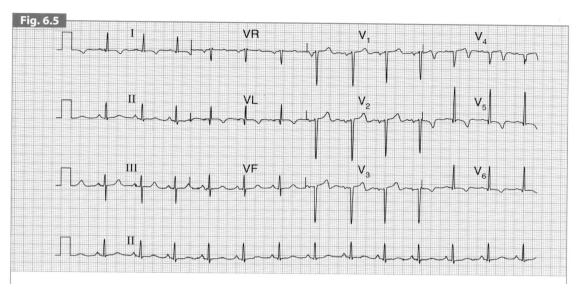

Old anterior ST segment elevation myocardial infarction

Note

- Sinus rhythm, rate 80/min
- Normal axis
- Q waves in leads VL and V_2–V_4
- Isoelectric (i.e. at baseline) ST segments (except in lead V_4)
- Inverted T waves in leads I, VL and V_4–V_6

135

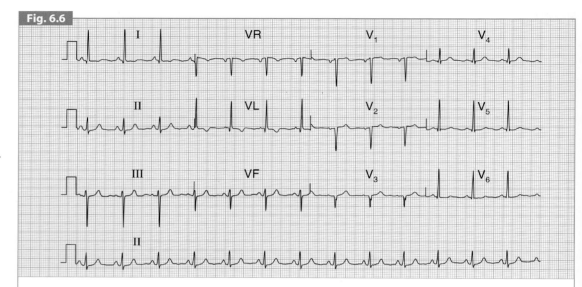

Fig. 6.6

Old anterior myocardial infarction with poor R wave progression in the anterior leads

Note

- Sinus rhythm, rate 80/min
- Normal axis (dominant S wave in lead III, but predominantly upright complex in leads I and II)
- Isoelectric ST segments
- The normal steady progression of R wave development in the anterior leads is missing, with no R wave in lead V_3 but a normal R wave in lead V_4
- Small Q wave and inverted T wave in lead VL
- This pattern might be due to inaccurate placement of the V_3 electrode, though the abnormal pattern in lead VL suggests cardiac disease. The ECG should be repeated

Fig. 6.7

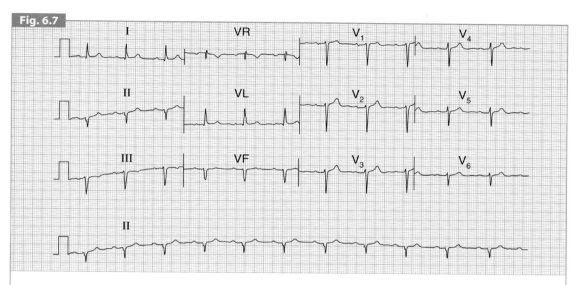

Clockwise rotation in chronic lung disease

Note

- Sinus rhythm, rate 70/min
- First degree block – PR interval 226 ms
- Left anterior hemiblock (predominantly downward complexes in leads II and III)
- QRS complexes show a 'right ventricular' pattern throughout, with a small R wave and a deep S wave in lead V_6, where there should be a tall R wave and a small S wave
- The first degree block and left anterior hemiblock indicate that cardiac disease is present, as well as chronic lung disease

Figures 6.8–6.10 are ECGs from a patient recorded a few hours after the onset of chest pain and a few days later, and they show the patterns of inferior infarction. Figure 6.8 shows a classic inferior STEMI, with, in addition, T wave inversion in lead VL. A few days later (Fig. 6.9), Q waves have appeared in leads III and VF, the ST segments have reverted almost

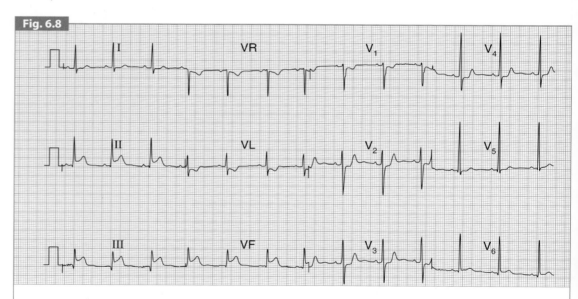

Fig. 6.8

Acute inferior ST segment elevation myocardial infarction

Note

- Sinus rhythm, rate 70/min
- Normal axis
- Small Q wave in lead III: other QRS complexes are normal
- ST segment elevation of 3 mm in leads II, III and VF
- T waves inverted in lead VL

to the baseline, and the T wave in lead VL is no longer inverted. During the acute phase of an inferior STEMI, conduction disturbances are quite common, as exemplified by the second degree block in Figure 6.10, showing the rhythm strip of an ECG recorded a few hours after that shown in Figure 6.8.

Fig. 6.9

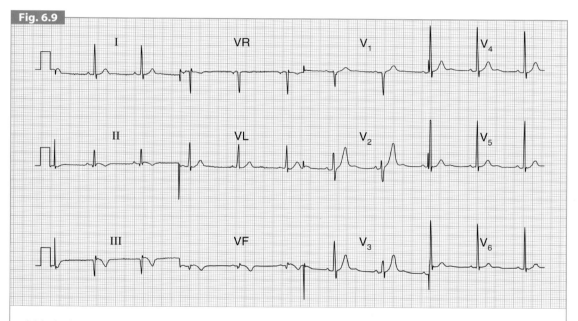

Old inferior myocardial infarction (same patient as in Figs 6.8 and 6.9)

Note
- Sinus rhythm, rate 60/min
- Normal axis
- Q waves in leads III and VF
- ST segments in leads II, III and VF have nearly returned to the baseline
- T waves inverted in leads II, III and VF
- QRS complexes and T waves are normal in the anterior leads

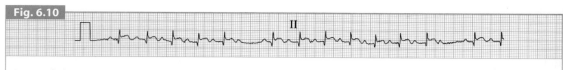

Fig. 6.10

Second degree (Wenckebach) heart block in inferior myocardial infarction (same patient as in Fig. 6.8)

Note
- Recorded from a monitor lead
- Sinus rhythm
- Progressive lengthening of the PR interval in the first few beats, followed by a nonconducted P wave, and then a similar sequence

For more on STEMI, see pp. 214–240

When an infarction develops in the posterior wall of the left ventricle, Q waves can only be elicited by placing the chest lead on the patient's back. In a routine ECG there will be a dominant R wave in lead V_1, caused by unopposed anterior depolarization (Fig. 6.11). This pattern must be differentiated from the dominant R wave in lead V_1 seen in pulmonary hypertension (see below), and from the dominant R wave that can be a normal variant. Differentiation is best made in the light of the patient's history and the physical findings.

140

Fig. 6.11

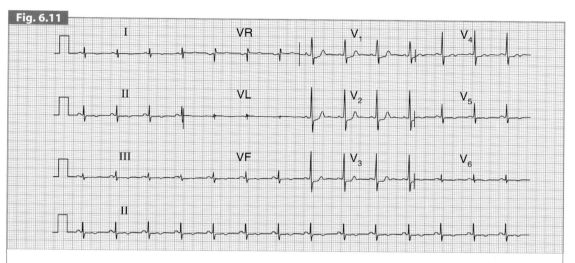

Old posterior myocardial infarction

Note

- Sinus rhythm, rate 85/min
- Dominant R wave in lead V$_1$
- ST segment depression in leads V$_1$–V$_3$
- T wave inversion in leads II, III, VF and V$_5$–V$_6$
- This pattern might be confused with a normal variant, or with right ventricular hypertrophy, but the ST segment and T wave changes suggest ischaemia, and there is no right axis deviation as would be expected with right ventricular hypertrophy

---

REMINDERS

STEMI

Sequence of ECG changes	**Site of infarction**
1. Normal ECG.	● Anterior infarction: changes classically in leads V_3–V_4, but often also in leads V_2 and V_5.
2. Raised ST segments.	● Inferior infarction: changes in leads III and VF.
3. Appearance of Q waves.	● Lateral infarction: changes in leads I, VL and V_5–V_6.
4. Normalization of ST segments.	● True posterior infarction: dominant R waves in lead V_1.
5. Inversion of T waves.	

NSTEMI

In NSTEMI there is no ST segment elevation, but there is T wave inversion in the leads corresponding to the site of myocardial damage (Fig. 6.12). With time the T waves may revert to normal, but inversion may persist. Q waves do not develop, and for this reason a distinction used to be made between 'Q wave' and 'non-Q wave' infarction. On the whole, Q-wave infarctions are STEMIs and non-Q wave infarctions are NSTEMIs. However, there is now treatment (PCI or thrombolysis) that can prevent Q wave development in a STEMI, making the Q/non-Q differentiation redundant.

Fig. 6.12

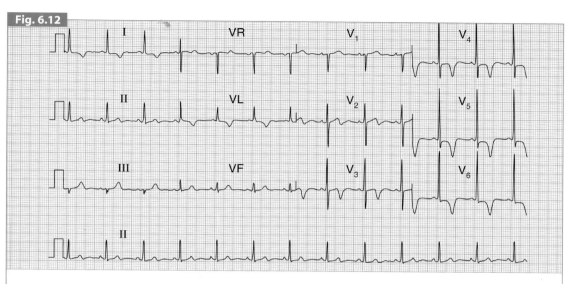

Anterior non-ST segment elevation myocardial infarction

Note

- Sinus rhythm, rate 75/min
- Normal axis
- Normal QRS complexes and ST segments
- T wave inversion in leads I, VL and V_3–V_6
- This pattern must be differentiated from that of left ventricular hypertrophy, where it would be most unusual to see T wave inversion in leads V_3–V_4

THE ECG IN PATIENTS WITH INTERMITTENT CHEST PAIN

Patients with angina may have a normal ECG when they are pain-free, although frequently the ECG shows evidence of a previous infarction. Patients whose chest pain is due to oesophageal disease or to muscular disorders, or whose pain is 'nonspecific', will also have a normal ECG.

In angina the ST segment typically becomes depressed, but when the angina is due to coronary vasospasm the ST segment may become elevated ('Prinzmetal's variant angina'). If a diagnosis of angina is in doubt, ECG changes can be induced by exercise. Exercise testing is less sensitive than, and is now being replaced by, stress echocardiography (and in some cardiologists' minds by immediate coronary angiography). However, exercise testing still has an important role in demonstrating a patient's tolerance to exercise, and in finding out just what limits him or her. Exercise testing has great advantages over coronary angiography: it is noninvasive, and the detection of coronary lesions during angiography does not necessarily mean that they are responsible for the patient's symptoms.

Exercise testing can be performed on a treadmill or an exercise bicycle, the former being more commonly used in the UK. After recording the ECG at rest, exercise is progressively increased in stages of 3 min. The most commonly used protocol is that devised by Bruce (Table 6.1). The two low-level stages (the 'modified Bruce protocol'), both at 2.7 kph but

Table 6.1 **Bruce protocol**

Stage	Speed (kph)	Speed (mph)	Gradient (degrees)
01	2.7	1.7	0
02	2.7	1.7	5
1	2.7	1.7	10
2	4.0	2.5	12
3	5.4	3.4	14
4	6.7	4.2	16
5	8.0	5.0	18

with a 0% or 5% gradient, can be used when a patient's exercise tolerance is markedly limited.

The heart rate, blood pressure and 12-lead ECG are recorded at the end of each stage. Exercise is continued until the patient asks to stop, but the test is ended early if the systolic blood pressure falls by more than 20 mmHg or the heart rate falls by more than 10/min. The test should also be ended if the patient develops chest pain and the ST segment in any lead is depressed by 2 mm, or if it is depressed by more than 3 mm without chest pain. The onset of any conduction disturbance or arrhythmia is also an indication for immediate discontinuation.

A diagnosis of cardiac ischaemia can confidently be made if there is horizontal ST segment depression of at least 2 mm. If the ST segments are depressed but upward-sloping, there is probably no ischaemia. Figures 6.13 and 6.14 show the ECG of a patient at rest and after exercise causing angina.

ECG
IP
For more on exercise testing, see pp. 270–284

Fig. 6.13

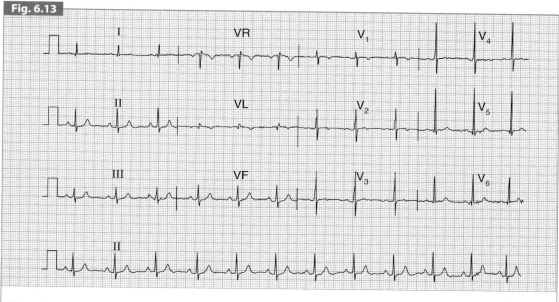

At rest

Note

- Sinus rhythm, rate 65/min
- Normal axis
- Normal QRS complexes, ST segments and T waves

Fig. 6.14

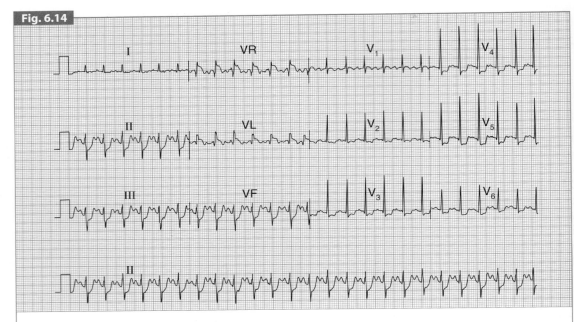

After 5 min of exercise (same patient as in Fig. 6.13)

Note

- Sinus rhythm, rate 150/min
- Left axis deviation
- Horizontal ST segment depression in the inferior and anterior leads, with a maximum of 4 mm in lead V_5

146

THE ECG IN PATIENTS WITH BREATHLESSNESS

Some causes of breathlessness are summarized in Box 6.3.

BREATHLESSNESS DUE TO HEART DISEASE

Remember that, although no particular ECG pattern corresponds to heart failure, this condition is unlikely with a completely normal ECG – other explanations for breathlessness should be considered. ECG evidence of cardiac enlargement may point to the cause of breathlessness. For example, ECG evidence of left ventricular hypertrophy may be due to hypertension or to mitral or aortic valve disease.

Box 6.3 **Causes of breathlessness**

- Lack of physical fitness
- Obesity
- Heart failure
- Lung disease
- Anaemia
- Neuromuscular disorders
- Chest wall pain

When the ECG of a breathless patient shows an arrhythmia or a conduction abnormality, or evidence of ischaemia or of atrial or ventricular hypertrophy, then the breathlessness may be due to heart failure.

REMINDERS
CARDIAC HYPERTROPHY

Right atrial hypertrophy
- Peaked P waves.

Right ventricular hypertrophy
- Tall R waves in lead V_1.
- T wave inversion in leads V_1 and V_2, and sometimes in V_3 and even V_4.
- Deep S waves in lead V_6.
- Right axis deviation.
- Sometimes, right bundle branch block.

Left atrial hypertrophy
- Bifid P waves.

Left ventricular hypertrophy
- R waves in lead V_5 or V_6 greater than 25 mm.
- R waves in lead V_5 or V_6 plus S waves in lead V_1 or V_2 greater than 35 mm.
- Inverted T waves in leads I, VL, V_5–V_6 and, sometimes, V_4.

BREATHLESSNESS DUE TO LUNG DISEASE

Pulmonary embolism

Pulmonary embolism often presents as a combination of chest pain and breathlessness. Although the chest pain is characteristically one-sided and pleuritic, a major embolus affecting the main pulmonary arteries may cause pain resembling that of myocardial infarction. Patients with pulmonary hypertension usually complain of breathlessness but not pain.

With pulmonary embolism the most common ECG finding is sinus tachycardia with no other abnormality (Fig. 6.15), so the ECG is not a very useful diagnostic tool. However, the appearance of right bundle branch block, or the changes associated with right ventricular hypertrophy (right axis deviation, a dominant R wave in lead V_1, and T wave inversion in leads V_1–V_3) would strongly support the diagnosis. If the patient develops permanent pulmonary hypertension, the full ECG picture of right ventricular hypertrophy will persist.

The commonly quoted 'S1Q3T3' pattern (i.e. right axis deviation with a prominent S wave in lead I and a Q wave and an inverted T wave in lead III) is seen in Figure 6.15, and is commonly quoted as an indicator of pulmonary embolism. In practice, it is not a very reliable indicator unless it is seen to appear in repeated recordings.

For more on pulmonary embolism, see pp. 247–250

REMINDERS

PULMONARY EMBOLISM

Possible ECG patterns include:

- Normal ECG with sinus tachycardia
- Peaked P waves
- Right axis deviation
- Right bundle branch block
- Dominant R waves in lead V_1 (i.e. R wave bigger than S wave)
- Inverted T waves in leads V_1–V_3
- Deep S waves in lead V_6
- Right axis deviation (S waves in lead I), plus Q waves and inverted T waves in lead III.

Fig. 6.15

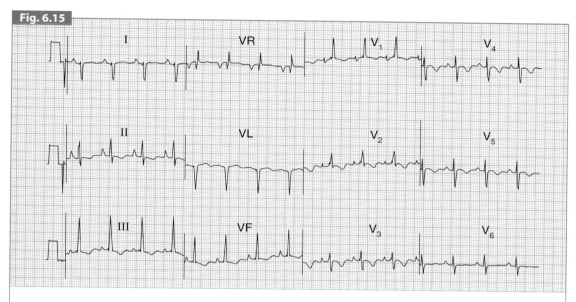

Pulmonary embolism

Note

- Sinus rhythm, rate 95/min
- Right axis deviation (QRS complexes predominantly downward in lead I)
- Peaked P waves in lead II, suggesting right atrial hypertrophy
- Persistent S wave in lead V_6
- T waves inverted in leads V_1, V_5, II, III and VF
- Right bundle branch block pattern

149

Chronic lung disease

Chronic obstructive pulmonary disease, pulmonary fibrosis and other intrinsic lung diseases do not usually cause the ECG changes associated with severe pulmonary hypertension, but there may be right axis deviation and, more often, clockwise rotation of the heart (Fig. 6.16). This is because the heart is rotated, with the right ventricle occupying more of the precordium than usual.

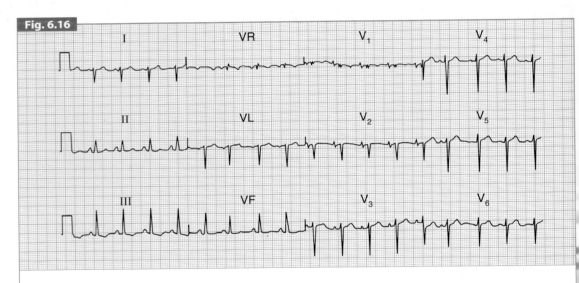

Fig. 6.16

Chronic lung disease

Note
- Sinus rhythm, rate 100/min
- Right axis deviation
- Peaked P waves, best seen in leads V_1–V_2
- Partial right bundle branch block
- Deep S waves in lead V_6, with no chest lead showing a pattern suggestive of left ventricular hypertrophy

The ECG in patients with palpitations or syncope

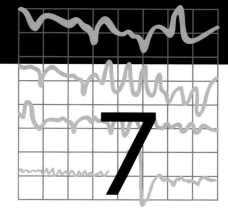

'Palpitations' means different things to different people, but essentially it means an awareness of the heartbeat. 'Syncope' means sudden loss of consciousness. The only way of being certain that a cardiac problem is the cause of either phenomenon is to record an ECG when the patient is having a typical attack, but this is seldom possible. Nevertheless, the ECG can be helpful, even when the patient is well.

THE ECG WHEN THE PATIENT HAS NO SYMPTOMS

If a patient is well at the time of recording, four possible ECG patterns can point to a diagnosis:

- Normal
- Patterns suggesting cardiac disease
- Patterns suggesting paroxysmal tachycardia
- Patterns suggesting syncope due to bradycardia.

NORMAL ECGs

Symptoms may not be due to heart disease – the patient may have epilepsy or some other condition. However, a normal ECG does not rule out a paroxysmal arrhythmia, and the patient's description of his or her symptoms may be crucial. For example, if the patient's attacks are associated with exercise (think of anaemia) or anxiety, and the palpitations build up and slow down, sinus tachycardia is likely to be the cause of the symptoms. In paroxysmal tachycardia, the attack begins suddenly, often for no obvious reason, and may stop suddenly. Ambulatory recording over 24 h, using, for example, the Holter technique, may be necessary to obtain a record of an attack (Fig. 7.1).

PATTERNS SUGGESTING CARDIAC DISEASE

Marked T wave inversion may suggest either left ventricular hypertrophy or left bundle branch block, which may be due to aortic stenosis; or right ventricular hypertrophy, which may be

due to pulmonary hypertension. In a young person, who is unlikely to have coronary disease, this pattern pattern suggests hypertrophic cardiomyopathy (Fig. 7.2), which is associated with arrhythmias, syncope and sudden death.

PATTERNS SUGGESTING PAROXYSMAL TACHYCARDIA

Pre-excitation syndromes

A PR interval that is short (less than 120 ms), with a wide and abnormal QRS complex, indicates the Wolff–Parkinson–White (WPW) syndrome. A short PR interval with a normal QRS complex suggests the Lown–Ganong–Levine (LGL) syndrome. In both cases an abnormal pathway bypasses the atrioventricular (AV) node, causing the short PR interval.

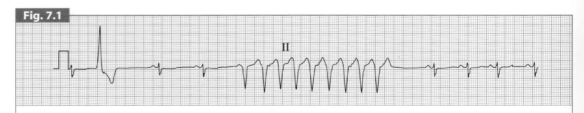

Fig. 7.1

II

Ambulatory recording: broad complex tachycardia

Note
- Ambulatory records provide only one or two leads, showing rhythm strips
- Sinus rhythm, rate 80/min
- One ventricular extrasystole
- A nine-beat run of broad complex tachycardia, probably ventricular in origin

Fig. 7.2

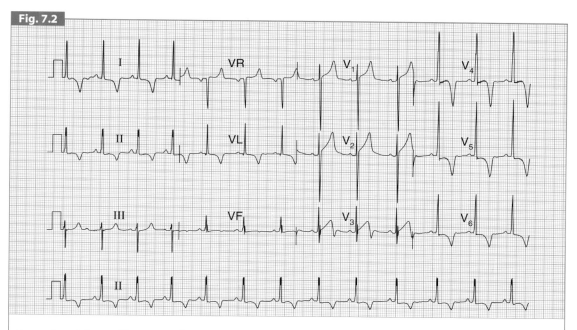

Hypertrophic cardiomyopathy

Note
- Sinus rhythm, rate 70/min
- Normal axis
- Left ventricular hypertrophy on voltage criteria (S wave in lead V_1 = 28 mm, R wave in lead V_5 = 30 mm)
- Deep T wave inversion in leads I, II, VL and V_3–V_6, maximal in lead V_4
- This ECG could be due to left ventricular hypertrophy rather than hypertrophic cardiomyopathy, but the T wave inversion is dramatic and is maximal in lead V_4 rather than in V_6. Anterolateral ischaemia is also unlikely, because of the marked nature of the T wave inversion

In the WPW syndrome, the abnormal pathway connects the atrium and the ventricle, and the QRS complex is wide, with a slurred upstroke. In the WPW syndrome type A, the pathway is left-sided, connecting the left atrium and left ventricle, and causes a dominant R wave in lead V_1 (Fig. 7.3; for another example see Fig. 3.28). This may be confused with right ventricular hypertrophy. Less commonly, the abnormal pathway can be right-sided, connecting the right atrium and right ventricle, and this is called the WPW syndrome type B (Fig. 7.4). Here, lead V_1 has no dominant R wave but has a deep S wave,

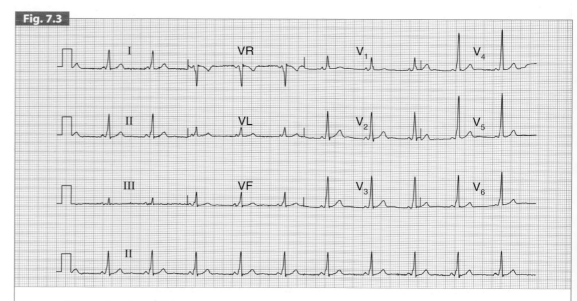

Fig. 7.3

The Wolff–Parkinson–White syndrome type A

Note
- Sinus rhythm, rate 65/min
- Normal axis
- Short PR interval (100 ms)
- QRS complexes slightly prolonged, at 130 ms; upstroke is slurred (best seen in leads V_4–V_5)
- Dominant R wave in lead V_1

Fig. 7.4

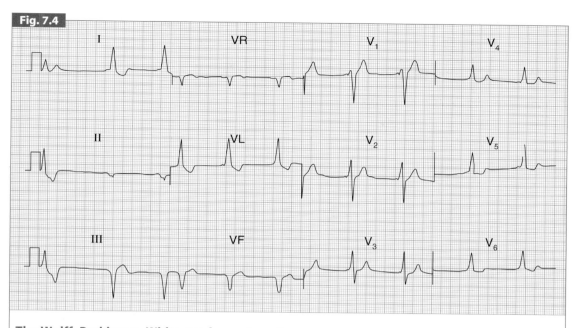

The Wolff–Parkinson–White syndrome type B

Note

- Sinus rhythm, rate 55/min – P waves best seen in lead V_1
- The first complex is probably a ventricular extrasystole
- Short PR interval
- Left axis deviation
- Broad QRS complexes (160 ms) with a slurred upstroke (delta wave), seen best in leads V_2–V_4
- Inverted T waves in leads I, II and VL, and biphasic T waves in leads V_5–V_6
- The small second and third complexes in lead II appear to be due to a technical error
- This record must be distinguished from sinus rhythm with left bundle branch block, and from the Wolff–Parkinson–White syndrome type A

and there is anterior T wave inversion, which may lead to a mistaken diagnosis of anterior ischaemia. The wide QRS complex seen in both types of the WPW syndrome may also lead to a mistaken diagnosis of bundle branch block, although the characteristic 'M' pattern of the QRS complexes in left bundle branch block is not seen in the WPW syndrome.

In the LGL syndrome the abnormal pathway connects the atria to the His bundle, so there is a short PR interval but a normal QRS complex (Fig. 7.5).

Fig. 7.5

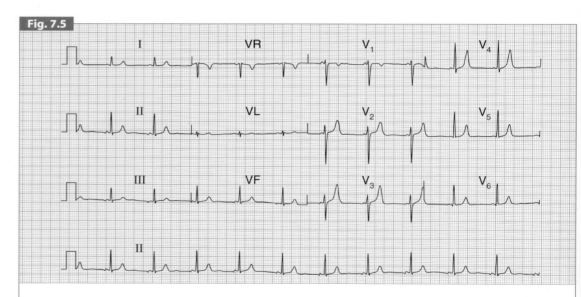

The Lown–Ganong–Levine syndrome

Note
- Sinus rhythm, rate 65/min
- Normal axis
- Short PR interval, 100 ms
- Normal QRS complexes and T waves
- In the LGL syndrome the accessory pathway connects the atria to the His bundle rather than to the right or left ventricle, so the QRS complex is normal

Long QT interval

The QT interval varies with the heart rate (and also with gender and the time of day). The corrected interval (QT$_c$) can be calculated using Bazett's formula:

$$QT_c = \frac{QT}{\sqrt{(R-R\ interval)}}$$

A QT$_c$ interval longer than 450 ms is likely to be abnormal. QT interval prolongation can be congenital, but is most often due to drugs, particularly to antiarrhythmic drugs (Box 7.1 and Fig. 7.6).

Whatever its cause, a corrected QT interval of 500 ms or longer can predispose to paroxysmal ventricular tachycardia of a particular type called 'torsade de pointes', which can cause either symptoms typical of paroxysmal tachycardia or sudden death. Figure 7.7 shows a continuous ECG from a patient who was being treated with an antiarrhythmic drug and who developed ventricular fibrillation while being monitored. A few seconds before the cardiac arrest, he developed a transient broad complex tachycardia in which the QRS complexes were initially upright but then changed, to become downward-pointing. This is typical of 'torsade de pointes' ventricular tachycardia.

Box 7.1 Causes of prolonged QT interval

Congenital
- Jervell–Lange–Nielson syndrome
- Romano–Ward syndrome
- Several other genetic abnormalities also identified

Antiarrhythmic drugs
- Procainamide
- Disopyramide
- Amiodarone
- Sotalol

Other drugs
- Tricyclic antidepressants
- Erythromycin

Plasma electrolyte abnormalities
- Low potassium
- Low magnesium
- Low calcium

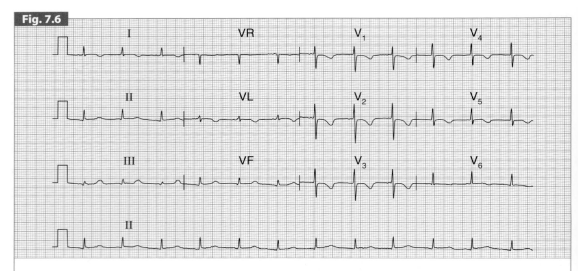

Fig. 7.6

Prolonged QT interval

Note

- Sinus rhythm, rate 75/min
- Normal axis
- P wave difficult to see in some leads, but most obvious in leads I and VL
- Normal QRS complexes
- T wave inversion in leads I, VL and V_1–V_6
- QT interval 480 ms, QT_c interval 520 ms
- In this patient the prolonged QT interval was due to amiodarone

Fig. 7.7

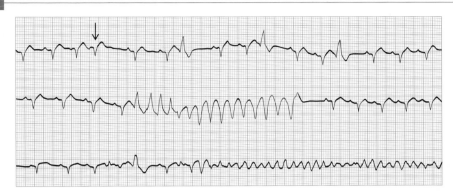

Torsade de pointes ventricular tachycardia and ventricular fibrillation

Note

- The three rhythm strips are a continuous record
- The underlying rhythm is sinus, rate about 100/min
- In the top strip there are one supraventricular extrasystole (arrowed) and three ventricular extrasystoles
- In the second strip there is a run of broad complex tachycardia, with the first four QRS complexes pointing upwards and the reminder pointing downwards – this is typical of torsade de pointes tachycardia
- In the bottom strip there is a single ventricular extrasystole and then ventricular fibrillation develops
- In this record a prolonged QT interval is not obvious – the QT interval is best measured on a 12-lead ECG

Sinoatrial disease

Sinoatrial disease, known as the 'sick sinus' syndrome, typically causes an inappropriate sinus bradycardia but is often asymptomatic (Fig. 7.8). It can also be associated with a variety of conduction problems, escape rhythms or paroxysmal tachycardia (Box 7.2). Patients may therefore complain of either dizziness, syncope or symptoms suggesting paroxysmal tachycardia.

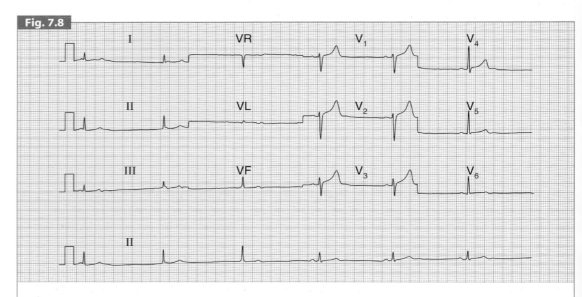

Fig. 7.8

Sick sinus syndrome

Note
- Look at the rhythm strip first
- The first three beats are due to AV nodal escape, with a rate of 35/min
- P waves can be seen immediately before or immediately after the QRS complex
- The next three beats are in sinus rhythm, rate 38/min
- The QRS complexes and T waves are normal
- A combination of sinus bradycardia and AV nodal escape is typical of the sick sinus syndrome

Box 7.2 Cardiac rhythms associated with sick sinus syndrome

- Inappropriate sinus bradycardia
- Sudden changes in the sinus rate
- Sinus pauses
- Atrial standstill
- Atrioventricular junctional escape rhythms
- Junctional tachycardia alternating with junctional escape

Box 7.3 Causes of heart block

First and second degree block
- Increased vagal tone
- Athletes
- Acute myocarditis
- Ischaemic heart disease
- Hypokalaemia
- Digoxin
- Beta-blockers

Complete block
- Idiopathic (fibrosis of conduction tissue)
- Congenital
- Ischaemic heart disease
- Aortic stenosis
- Surgery and trauma

PATTERNS SUGGESTING SYNCOPE DUE TO BRADYCARDIA

In apparently healthy subjects who complain of attacks of dizziness, the resting ECG when asymptomatic may show axis deviation, sick sinus syndrome or any variety of heart block. First degree block, second degree block of the Wenckebach (Mobitz type 1) variety, and bundle branch block do not in themselves indicate treatment, and neither do combinations of these blocks, such as first degree block and bundle branch block (Fig. 7.9), or bifascicular block (left anterior hemiblock and right bundle branch block, Fig. 7.10). However, such combinations may also be associated with higher degrees of block, and ambulatory recording may be considered to see if second or third degree block is occurring intermittently.

In a patient with second degree block (Mobitz type 2, 2:1 block or 3:1 block) or complete (third degree) block, it is likely that any dizziness or syncope is due to a low heart rate, and pacing is indicated without the need for ambulatory recording first.

It is important to consider the possible underlying causes of heart block, and these are summarized in Box 7.3.

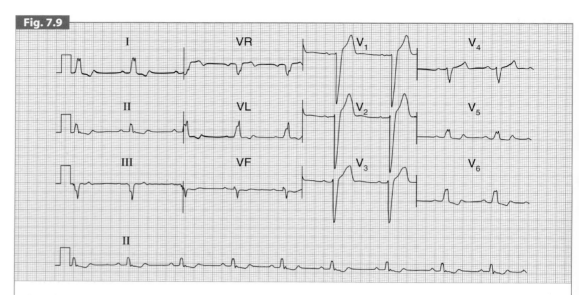

Fig. 7.9

First degree block and left bundle branch block

Note
- Sinus rhythm, rate 55/min
- Normal axis
- Prolonged PR interval, 224 ms
- Wide QRS complexes
- 'M' pattern in leads I, II, V$_5$ and V$_6$
- Inverted T waves in leads I, VL and V$_6$

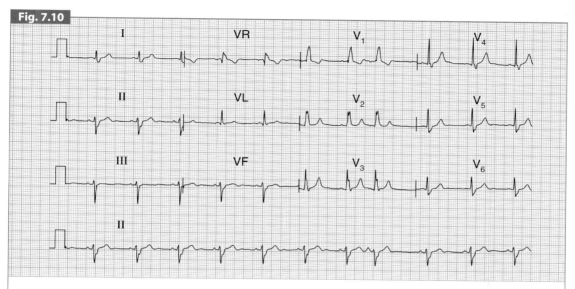

Fig. 7.10

Bifascicular block

Note

- Sinus rhythm, rate 70/min
- Left axis deviation (S wave greater than R wave in leads II and III)
- Right bundle branch block – wide QRS complexes (135 ms); RSR[1] pattern in lead V_1; and a wide slurred S wave in lead V_6

THE ECG WHEN THE PATIENT HAS SYMPTOMS

PAROXYSMAL TACHYCARDIA

It is not possible to tell from a patient's symptoms whether extrasystoles or a paroxysmal tachycardia are supraventricular or ventricular in origin – although paroxysmal ventricular tachycardia is perhaps more likely to cause dizziness or syncope than paroxysmal supraventricular tachycardia.

In a paroxysmal tachycardia, the heart rate is usually greater than 160/min – compared with sinus tachycardia, in which it is seldom greater than 140/min. The QRS complexes in paroxysmal tachycardia can be narrow (i.e. less than 120 ms) or broad.

Narrow complex tachycardias may indicate:

- Sinus tachycardia
- Atrial tachycardia
- Junctional (AV nodal re-entry) tachycardia
- Atrial flutter
- Atrial fibrillation
- The WPW syndrome.

The ECG characteristics of the supraventricular rhythms are summarized in the Reminders on page 165.

The simplest way to identify the cause of narrow complex tachycardia is to apply carotid sinus pressure while recording an ECG. This will cause sinus tachycardia to slow; atrial and junctional tachycardias and tachycardias due to pre-excitation may be abolished; in atrial flutter the atrioventricular block will increase; and

atrial fibrillation will not usually be affected (see p. 72).

Broad complex tachycardias indicate:

- Ventricular tachycardia
- Supraventricular tachycardia of any type (other than sinus rhythm) with bundle branch block
- The WPW syndrome.

REMINDERS
THE VENTRICULAR RHYTHMS

- In general, ventricular rhythms have wide (greater than 120 ms) QRS complexes; a change of axis compared to sinus rhythm; and abnormal T waves.
- Ventricular extrasystoles:
  - early QRS complex
  - no P wave
  - QRS complex wide (greater than 120 ms)
  - abnormally shaped QRS complex
  - abnormally shaped T wave
  - next P wave is on time.
- Accelerated idioventricular rhythm:
  - no P wave
  - QRS rate less than 120/min.
- Ventricular tachycardia:
  - no P waves
  - QRS rate greater than 160/min.
- Ventricular fibrillation:
  - look at the patient, not at the ECG.

The ECG characteristics of the broad complex tachycardias are summarized in the Reminders on page 164.

It can be very difficult to differentiate between the broad complexes of a supraventricular tachycardia with bundle

---

REMINDERS

THE SUPRAVENTRICULAR RHYTHMS

- In general, supraventricular rhythms have narrow (less than 120 ms) QRS complexes, the exceptions being bundle branch block and the WPW syndrome, in which wide QRS complexes are seen.
- Sinus rhythm:
  - one P wave per QRS complex
  - P–P interval varies with respiration (sinus arrhythmia).
- Supraventricular extrasystoles:
  - early QRS complex
  - no P wave, or abnormally shaped (atrial) P wave
  - narrow and normal QRS complex
  - normal T wave
  - next P wave is 'reset'.
- Atrial tachycardia:
  - QRS complex rate greater than 150/min
  - abnormal P waves, usually with short PR intervals
  - usually one P wave per QRS complex, but sometimes P wave rate 200–240/min, with 2:1 block.

- Atrial flutter:
  - P wave rate 300/min
  - sawtoothed pattern
  - 2:1, 3:1 or 4:1 block
  - block increased by carotid sinus pressure.
- Atrial fibrillation:
  - the most irregular rhythm of all
  - QRS complex rate characteristically over 160/min without treatment, but can be slower
  - no P waves identifiable, but there is a varying, completely irregular baseline.
- AV nodal re-entry (junctional) tachycardia:
  - commonly, but inappropriately, called 'SVT' (supraventricular tachycardia)
  - no P waves
  - rate usually 150–180/min
  - carotid sinus pressure may cause reversion to sinus rhythm.
- Escape rhythms:
  - bradycardias, otherwise characteristics as above, except that atrial fibrillation does not occur as an escape rhythm.

branch block and ventricular tachycardia, but the following Reminders should help.

Figure 7.11 shows an ECG with all the usual features of ventricular tachycardia – left axis deviation, QRS complexes with duration 180 ms, and all the complexes in the chest leads pointing upwards.

REMINDERS

BROAD COMPLEX TACHYCARDIAS

- When seen in the context of acute myocardial infarction, a broad complex tachycardia is likely to be ventricular in origin.
- Comparison with a record made during sinus rhythm (if available) will show if bundle branch block is normally present.
- Try to identify P waves.
- Left axis deviation with right bundle branch block is usually indicates a ventricular problem.
- Very wide (greater than 160 ms) QRS complexes usually indicate ventricular tachycardia.
- Concordance – ventricular tachycardia is likely if the QRS complexes all point predominantly upwards or downwards in the chest leads.
- An irregular broad complex rhythm is likely to be atrial fibrillation with bundle branch block, or atrial fibrillation in the WPW syndrome (a dangerous combination).

INTERMITTENT BRADYCARDIA

Intermittent bradycardia due to any cardiac rhythm can cause dizziness and syncope if the heart rate is low enough. Athletes can be perfectly healthy with a sinus rate of 40/min, but an elderly person may become dizzy if the heart rate drops below 60/min for any reason.

A low rate can be due to second or third degree heart block (see pp. 37–42) or to 'pauses', when the sinoatrial node fails to depolarize. This is seen in the sick sinus syndrome. Figure 7.12 shows an ambulatory record from a patient with sick sinus syndrome, who complained of attacks of dizziness which were due to sinus pauses of 3.3 s.

There is no effective medical treatment for symptomatic bradycardia, and permanent pacing may be necessary.

In the context of acute myocardial infarction, particularly inferior ST segment elevation myocardial infarction (STEMI), complete heart block is not uncommon. It is usually temporary, and does not need pacing unless there is haemodynamic impairment due to a slow heart rate. When complete block complicates an anterior STEMI, a large amount of myocardium has usually been damaged, and temporary pacing may be needed.

Fig. 7.11

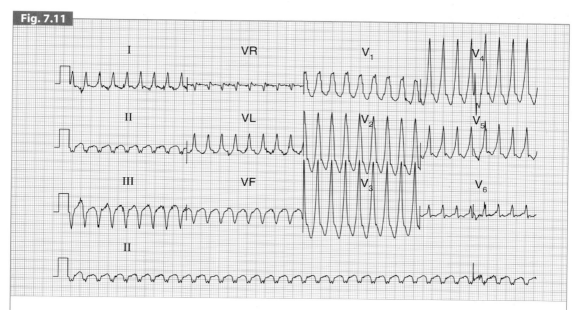

Ventricular tachycardia

Note

- Regular broad complex tachycardia, rate 200/min
- No P waves visible
- Left axis deviation
- QRS complex duration 180 ms (if >160 ms, the rhythm is more likely to be ventricular in origin than to be supraventricular with bundle branch block)
- QRS complexes all point the same way (upwards) in the chest leads (again, makes a ventricular origin likely)

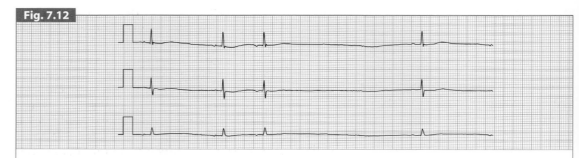

Fig. 7.12

Ambulatory record, sick sinus syndrome

Note
- The first two beats demonstrate sinus rhythm, rate 38/min
- The third beat is an atrial extrasystole, shown by an abnormal P wave
- There is then a prolonged pause lasting 3.5 s, followed by another sinus beat

PACEMAKERS

Pacemakers produce a small electrical discharge that either replaces the function of the sinoatrial node or bypasses a blocked His bundle. The sophisticated design of pacemakers enables them to mimic many of the functions of the normal heart.

Pacemaker function can be assessed from the resting ECG. Most modern pacemakers sense the intrinsic activation of the atria and/or the ventricles, and may pace both. The operating mode of a pacemaker can be described in three or four letters:

1. The first letter describes the chamber(s) paced (A for right atrium, V for right ventricle or D for dual, i.e. both chambers).
2. The second letter describes the chambers sensed (A, V or D).
3. The third letter describes the response to a sensed event (A, V or D for pacing; I for pacemaker inhibition).
4. The fourth letter (R) is used when the rate modulation is programmable.

Thus, 'VVI' means that the pacemaker paces and senses the right ventricle. When no spontaneous activity is sensed, the pacemaker stimulates the right ventricle; and when spontaneous activity is sensed, the pacemaker is inhibited. The ECG looks like that in Figure 7.13.

'AAI' means that the pacemaker has a single lead in the atrium, to both sense and pace it (Fig. 7.14). If the pacemaker does not sense spontaneous atrial depolarization, it stimulates the atrium; and when there is spontaneous depolarization, the pacemaker is inhibited.

'DDD' means that there are pacemaker leads in both the right atrium and the right ventricle, and both chambers are sensed and paced. If no atrial activity is sensed within a predetermined period, the atrial pacing lead will pace. A maximum PR interval is also predetermined, and if no ventricular beat is sensed, the ventricle will be paced. Figure 7.13 could be the result of simple VVI pacing, or could be the result of atrial sensing and ventricular pacing, the ventricular rate 'following' the atrial rate. A chest X-ray would show whether there were one or two pacing leads. Figure 7.15 shows both atrial and ventricular pacing.

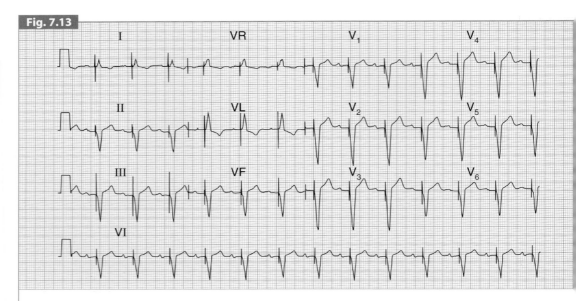

Fig. 7.13

Ventricular pacing

Note

- Ventricular paced rhythm: there is a sharp pacemaker spike before each QRS complex
- The QRS complexes are wide and abnormal
- Sinus rate, 75/min
- Prolonged PR interval, 280 ms
- Each paced beat follows a P wave
- This could be VVI pacing, but the pacemaker is probably tracking the atrial rate by means of a sensing catheter in the right atrium (DDD pacing)

Fig. 7.14

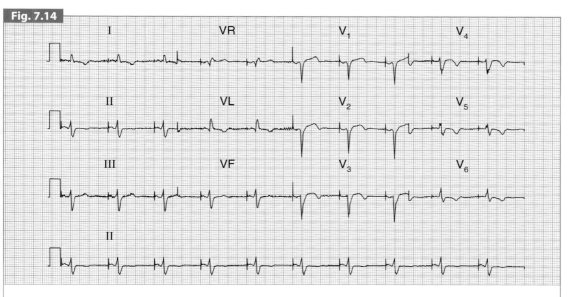

Atrial pacing

Note

- Atrial paced rhythm, shown by a sharp pacing spike immediately before each P wave
- Normal PR interval
- The QRS complexes are narrow but there is a lack of R wave development in the anterior leads, suggesting an old anterior infarction
- T waves inverted in leads II, VL and V_4–V_6, consistent with ischaemia
- In atrial pacing the QRS complexes and T waves can be interpreted, whereas in ventricular pacing they are bound to be abnormal

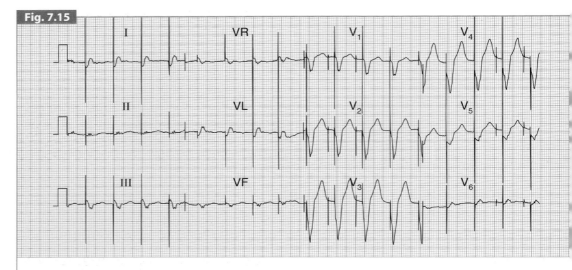

Fig. 7.15

Dual chamber pacing

Note
- Two pacing spikes can be seen, most clearly in leads V_1–V_3
- The first spike causes atrial activity, though no clear P wave can be seen
- The second spike causes ventricular activity, with a wide and abnormal QRS complex

CARDIAC ARREST

Cardiac arrest can be classified according to whether the rhythm is 'shockable' (i.e. correctable by DC cardioversion) or nonshockable. In either case, the first part of the treatment is a precordial thump and cardiopulmonary resuscitation at 30 compressions for each two ventilations.

The shockable rhythms are ventricular fibrillation (VF) and pulseless ventricular tachycardia (VT). Action in either case, following the first two steps, should be:

1. Precordial thump.
2. One shock at 200 J.
3. Resume chest compressions at 30:2 for 2 min, then check the rhythm.
4. If unsuccessful, defibrillate at 360 J.
5. If unsuccessful, give adrenaline 1 mg i.v.
6. Defibrillate at 360 J.
7. 2 min of cardiopulmonary rescuscitation (CPR).
8. If VF or pulseless VT persists, give amiodarone 300 mg i.v.
9. Give further shocks after 2-min periods of CPR, with adrenaline 1 mg i.v. before alternate shocks.
10. For refractory VF, give magnesium sulfate 2 g i.v. bolus (8 mmol).

Note that adrenaline is given intravenously only for cardiac arrest. When adrenaline is given for anaphylactic shock (the combination of laryngeal oedema, bronchospasm and hypotension), the dose is 0.5 mg given *intramuscularly*, because adrenaline given intravenously can cause cardiac arrhythmias.

The nonshockable rhythms are asystole and pulseless electrical activity (PEA). If it is not clear whether the rhythm is 'fine' VF or asystole, treat as VF until three defibrillations have not changed the apparent rhythm. The treatment sequence after the first two steps is:

1. Adrenaline 1 mg i.v.
2. CPR 30:2 for 2 min.
3. Atropine 3 mg i.v.
4. If unsuccessful, continue adrenaline 1 mg after alternate 2-min cycles of CPR.

Particularly in cases of PEA, consider possible reversible causes of cardiac arrest, all of which begin with H or T and are listed in Box 7.4.

Box 7.4 Causes of nonshockable rhythms

- Hypoxia
- Hypovolaemia
- Hyperkalaemia, hypokalaemia, hypocalcaemia, acidosis, hypoglycaemia
- Hypothermia
- Tamponade
- Tension pneumothorax
- Toxic substances, including drug overdoses
- Thromboembolism, e.g. pulmonary embolism

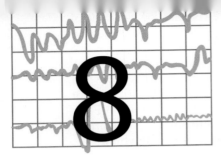

8

Now test yourself

You should now be able to recognize the common ECG patterns, and this final chapter contains ten 12-lead records for you to interpret. But do not forget two important things: first, an ECG comes from an individual patient and must be interpreted with the patient in mind, and second, there is little point in recording and interpreting an ECG unless you are prepared to take some action based on your findings. This is a theme developed in the companion to this book, *150 ECG Problems*.

When reporting an ECG, remember:

1. The ECG is easy.
2. A report has two parts – a description and an interpretation.

3. Look at all the leads, and describe the ECG in the same order every time:
   rate and rhythm
   – conduction
   – PR interval if sinus rhythm
   – cardiac axis
   – QRS complexes:
     ● duration
     ● height of R and S waves
     ● presence of Q waves
   – ST segments
   – T waves.
4. The range of normality, and especially which leads can show an inverted T wave in a normal ECG.

Only after carefully thinking about every aspect of the ECG pattern, and the patient's history, should you make a diagnosis. You may find the Reminders displayed below helpful.

REMINDERS

WHAT TO LOOK FOR

1. The rhythm and conduction:
   - sinus rhythm or some early arrhythmias
   - evidence of first, second or third degeree block
   - evidence of bundle branch block.
2. P wave abnormalities:
   - peaked, tall – right atrial hypertrophy
   - notched, broad – left atrial hypertrophy.
3. The cardiac axis:
   - right axis deviation – QRS complex predominantly downward in lead I
   - left axis deviation – QRS complex predominantly downward in leads II and III.
4. The QRS complex:
   - width:
     - if wide, ventricular origin, bundle branch block or the WPW syndrome
   - height:
     - tall R waves in lead V_1 in right ventricular hypertrophy
     - tall R waves in lead V_6 in left ventricular hypertrophy
   - transition point:
     - R and S waves are equal in the chest leads over the interventricular septum (normally lead V_3 or V_4)
     - clockwise rotation (persistent S wave in lead V_6) indicates chronic lung disease.

- Q waves:
  - ? septal
  - ? infarction.
5. The ST segment:
   - raised in acute myocardial infarction and in pericarditis
   - depressed in ischaemia and with digoxin.
6. T waves:
   - peaked in hyperkalaemia
   - flat, prolonged, in hypokalaemia
   - inverted:
     - normal in some leads
     - ischaemia
     - infarction
     - left or right ventricular hypertrophy
     - pulmonary embolism
     - bundle branch block.
7. U waves:
   - can be normal
   - hypokalaemia.

REMINDERS

CONDUCTION PROBLEMS

First degree block

- One P wave per QRS complex.
- PR interval greater than 200 ms.

Second degree block

- Wenckebach (Mobitz type 1): progressive PR lengthening then a nonconducted P wave, and then repetition of the cycle.
- Mobitz type 2: occasional nonconducted beats.
- 2:1 (or 3:1) block: two (or three) P waves per QRS complex, with a normal P wave rate.

Third degree (complete) block

- No relationship between P waves and QRS complexes.
- Usually, wide QRS complexes.
- Usual QRS complex rate less than 50/min.
- Sometimes, narrow QRS complexes, rate 50–60/min.

Right bundle branch block

- QRS complex duration greater than 120 ms.
- RSR^1 pattern.
- Usually, dominant R^1 wave in lead V_1.
- Inverted T waves in lead V_1, and sometimes in leads V_2–V_3.
- Deep and wide S waves in lead V_6.

Left anterior hemiblock

- Marked left axis deviation – deep S waves in leads II and III, usually with a slightly wide QRS complex.

Left bundle branch block

- QRS complex duration greater than 120 ms.
- 'M' pattern in lead V_6, and sometimes in leads V_4–V_5.
- No septal Q waves.
- Inverted T waves in leads I, VL, V_5–V_6 and, sometimes, V_4.

Bifascicular block

- Left anterior hemiblock and right bundle branch block (see above).

REMINDERS

CAUSES OF AXIS DEVIATION

Right axis deviation

- Normal variant – tall thin people.
- Right ventricular hypertrophy.
- Lateral myocardial infarction (peri-infarction block).
- Dextrocardia or right/left arm lead switch.
- The Wolff–Parkinson–White (WPW) syndrome.
- Left posterior fascicular block.

Left axis deviation

- Left anterior hemiblock.
- The WPW syndrome.
- Inferior myocardial infarction (peri-infarction block).
- Ventricular tachycardia.

REMINDERS

POSSIBLE IMPLICATIONS OF ECG PATTERNS

P:QRS apparently not 1:1

If you cannot see one P wave per QRS complex, consider the following:

- If the P wave is actually present but not easily visible, look particularly at leads II and V_1.
- If the QRS complexes are irregular, the rhythm is probably atrial fibrillation, and what seem to be P waves actually are not.
- If the QRS complex rate is rapid and there are no P waves, a wide QRS complex indicates ventricular tachycardia, and a narrow QRS complex indicates atrioventricular nodal (junctional or AV nodal) re-entry tachycardia.
- If the QRS complex rate is low, it is probably an escape rhythm.

P:QRS more than 1:1

If you can see more P waves than QRS complexes, consider the following:

- If the P wave rate is 300/min, the rhythm is atrial flutter.
- If the P wave rate is 150–200/min and there are two P waves per QRS complex, the rhythm is atrial tachycardia with block.
- If the P wave rate is normal (i.e. 60–100/min) and there is 2:1 conduction, the rhythm is sinus with second degree block.
- If the PR interval appears to be different with each beat, complete (third degree) heart block is probably present.

continued

REMINDERS
POSSIBLE IMPLICATIONS OF ECG PATTERNS – *continued*

Wide QRS complexes (greater than 120 ms)
Wide QRS complexes are characteristic of:

- Sinus rhythm with bundle branch block
- Sinus rhythm with the WPW syndrome
- Ventricular extrasystoles
- Ventricular tachycardia
- Complete heart block.

Q waves
- Small (septal) Q waves are normal in leads I, VL and V_6.
- A Q wave in lead III but not in VF is a normal variant.
- Q waves probably indicate infarction if present in more than one lead, are longer than 40 ms in duration and are deeper than 2 mm.
- Q waves in lead III but not in VF, plus right axis deviation, may indicate pulmonary embolism.
- The leads showing Q waves indicate the site of an infarction.

ST segment depression
- Digoxin: ST segment slopes downwards.
- Ischaemia: flat ST segment depression.

T wave inversion
- Normal in leads III, VR and V_1; and in V_2–V_3 in black people.
- Ventricular rhythms.
- Bundle branch block.
- Myocardial infarction.
- Right or left ventricular hypertrophy.
- The WPW syndrome.

ECGs WITH CLINICAL SCENARIOS

The following ECGs (1–10) are in no particular sequence, and similar ECGs have been described earlier in this book. With each there is a short clinical scenario, and their descriptions and interpretations commence on p. 185.

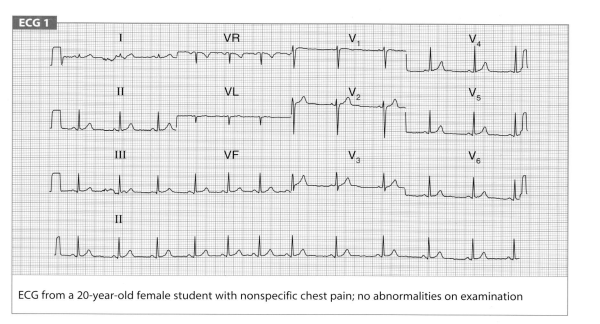

ECG 1

ECG from a 20-year-old female student with nonspecific chest pain; no abnormalities on examination

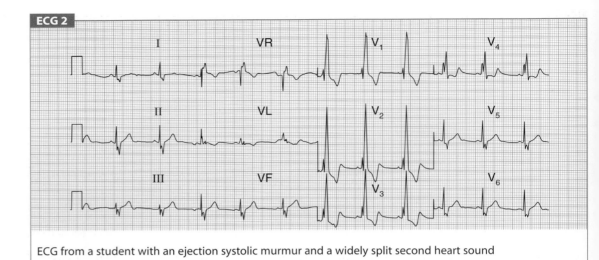

ECG from a student with an ejection systolic murmur and a widely split second heart sound

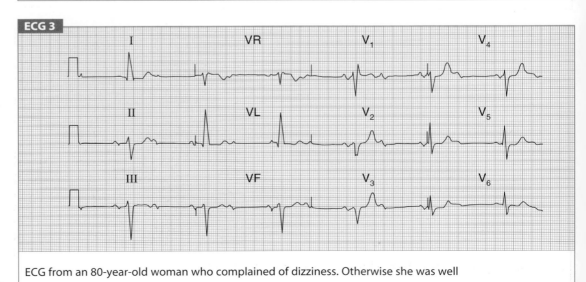

ECG from an 80-year-old woman who complained of dizziness. Otherwise she was well

ECG 4

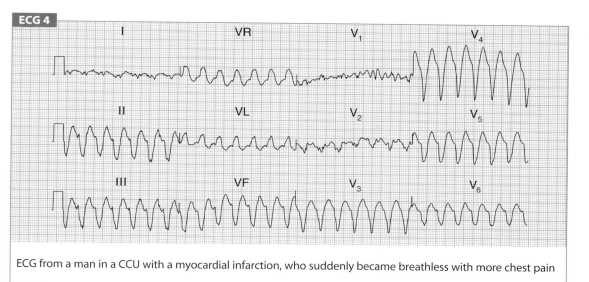

ECG from a man in a CCU with a myocardial infarction, who suddenly became breathless with more chest pain

ECG 5

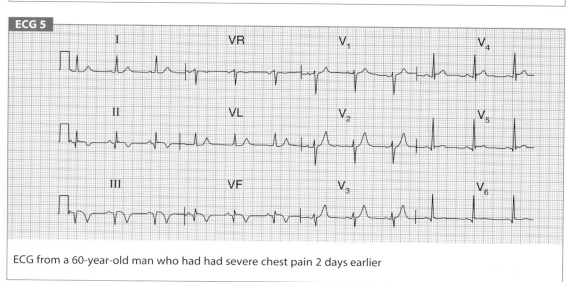

ECG from a 60-year-old man who had had severe chest pain 2 days earlier

181

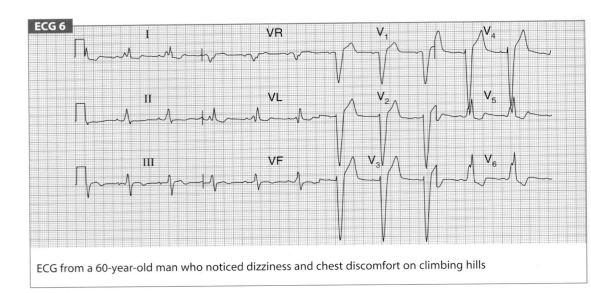

ECG 6

ECG from a 60-year-old man who noticed dizziness and chest discomfort on climbing hills

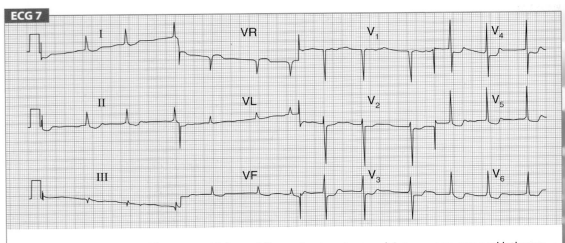

ECG 7

ECG from a small 70-year-old woman with heart failure, whose main complaints were nausea and lethargy

ECG 8

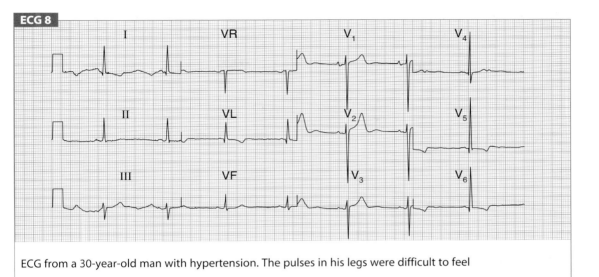

ECG from a 30-year-old man with hypertension. The pulses in his legs were difficult to feel

ECG 9

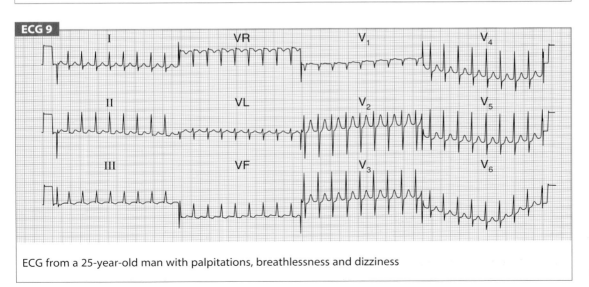

ECG from a 25-year-old man with palpitations, breathlessness and dizziness

ECG 10

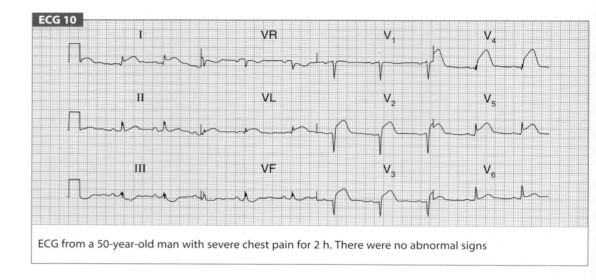

ECG from a 50-year-old man with severe chest pain for 2 h. There were no abnormal signs

ECG DESCRIPTIONS AND INTERPRETATIONS

ECG 1

This ECG shows:

- Sinus rhythm; the rhythm strip (lead II) shows sinus arrhythmia
- The heart rate change (most obvious in leads VF and V_3) is due to sinus arrhythmia
- Normal PR interval, 120 ms
- Normal axis
- QRS complex duration 80 ms, normal height
- ST segment isoelectric in all leads
- T wave inversion in lead VR, but no other lead.

Interpretation of the ECG

This is a perfectly normal record in all respects. The sinus arrhythmia is clearly shown in the section of the rhythm strip below: the change in the R–R interval is progressive from beat to beat. The configuration of the P wave does not change, so there is sinus rhythm throughout.

If you did not get this right, look at p. 32.

Clinical management

The description of the pain does not sound in the least cardiac, and a young woman is very unlikely to have coronary disease anyway. If you find yourself making a diagnosis on the basis of an ECG that seems clinically unlikely, think about the ECG a little further. This pain sounds muscular, and she only needs reassurance.

ECG 2

This ECG shows:

- Sinus rhythm
- Normal PR interval
- Normal axis
- Wide QRS complex duration, at 160 ms
- RSR^1 pattern in lead V_1
- Wide and notched S wave in lead V_6
- ST segment isoelectric
- T wave inversion in lead VR (normal), and in leads V_1–V_3.

Rhythm strip (ECG 1)

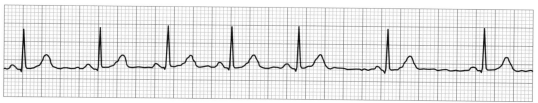

Interpretation of the ECG

There is no problem with conduction between the atria and the ventricles because the PR interval is normal and constant. The prolonged QRS complex duration shows that there is conduction delay within the ventricles. The RSR[1] pattern in lead V_1 and the deep and wide S wave in lead V_6 (see the extracts from the traces, below) are characteristic of right bundle branch block (RBBB).

Any problems? If so, look at pp. 44–45.

Clinical management

The story raises the possibility that this young woman has a congenital heart problem. Fixed wide splitting of the second heart sound is the clinical manifestation of RBBB, with which pulmonary valve closure is delayed. RBBB is characteristic of an atrial septal defect, and an

echocardiogram is essential to confirm the diagnosis and to help decide if, how and when it should be closed.

ECG 3

This ECG shows:

- Sinus rhythm
- Alternate conducted and nonconducted beats
- Normal PR interval in the conducted beats
- Left axis deviation (deep S waves in leads II and III)
- Wide QRS complex (duration 160 ms)
- RSR[1] pattern in lead V_1
- Note: the sharp spikes are due to lead changes, not to a pacemaker.

Interpretation of the ECG

The alternating conducted and nonconducted P waves indicate second degree heart block, and this explains the slow heart rate. The left axis deviation shows that conduction down the anterior fascicle of the left bundle branch is blocked, and the RSR[1] pattern in lead V_1 indicates RBBB (see the extracts from the traces, opposite page).

This was explained in Chapter 2.

Clinical management

This patient clearly has severe disease of her conduction system. Both bundle branches are affected, and the second degree block probably

ECG
IP

For more on congenital heart disease, see pp. 320–326

RSR[1] pattern and S wave (ECG 2)

V_1

V_6

Left axis deviation, RSR^1 pattern and P waves (ECG 3)

I

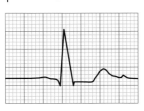

II

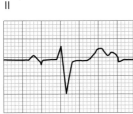

III

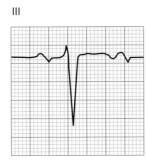

V$_1$

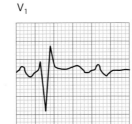

VL

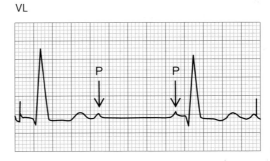

results from disease in the His bundle. The attacks of dizziness may be due to further slowing of the heart rate with the same rhythm, or may be due to intermittent complete heart block (Stokes–Adams attacks). This could be investigated with a 24-h ambulatory ECG recording, but this is not really necessary as she needs an immediate permanent pacemaker.

ECG
IP

For more on pacemakers, see pp. 187–206

ECG 4

This ECG shows:

- Broad complex tachycardia at 160/min
- No P waves visible
- Left axis deviation
- QRS complex duration 200 ms
- QRS complexes all point downwards in the chest leads
- Artefacts in leads I and V_1–V_2.

Interpretation of the ECG

The QRS complexes are broad, so this is either ventricular tachycardia or supraventricular tachycardia with bundle branch block. There are no P waves, so it is not sinus rhythm or an atrial rhythm. The QRS complexes are regular, so it is not atrial fibrillation, but an AV nodal rhythm with bundle branch block is a possibility. However, the left axis deviation, and the 'concordance' of the QRS complexes (all pointing downwards), makes this ventricular tachycardia (see the extracts from the traces, below).

For the diagnosis of tachycardias, see p. 75.

Clinical management

In the context of a myocardial infarction, broad complex tachycardia is almost always ventricular in origin, and there is no need to get too puzzled by the ECG. This patient has developed pulmonary oedema, so needs urgent treatment. While preparations are made for DC cardioversion, he could be given intravenous lidocaine and furosemide, but you should not rely on a satisfactory response to drug therapy.

ECG 5

This ECG shows:

- Sinus rhythm
- Normal PR interval
- Normal axis
- QRS complex has Q waves in leads II, III and VF
- ST segment isoelectric
- T waves inverted in leads II, III and VF.

ECG
IP

For more on differentiation of broad complex tachycardias, see p. 126

Left axis deviation and QRS complexes (ECG 4)

II

III

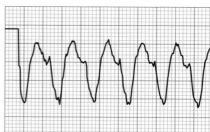

Interpretation of the ECG

The Q waves in leads III and VF, together with the inverted T waves in those leads (see the extract from the trace, below), indicate an inferior myocardial infarction. Since the ST segment is virtually isoelectric (i.e. at the baseline, and not elevated) the infarction is 'old'. The ECG can show this pattern at any time after the 24 h following the infarction, so timing the event is not possible from the ECG.
   Get this one wrong? Read pp. 91–96.

Clinical management

The clinical story suggests that the infarction occurred 48 h previously. This patient has presented too late for immediate treatment of the infarction by thrombolysis or urgent angioplasty, and he does not need pain relief or any treatment for complications. The aim of management is therefore to prevent a further infarction, and he will need long-term aspirin, a beta-blocker, an ACE (angiotensin-converting enzyme) inhibitor and a statin. He will also need an exercise test, and a decision will need to be made about the need for coronary angiography.

ECG 6

This ECG shows:

- Sinus rhythm
- Normal PR interval
- Normal axis
- Wide QRS complexes, duration 200 ms
- 'M' pattern in leads I, VL and V_5–V_6
- Deep S waves in leads V_2–V_4
- Biphasic or inverted T waves in leads I, VL and V_5–V_6

Interpretation of the ECG

The rhythm and PR interval are normal but the wide QRS complexes show that there is a conduction delay within the ventricles. The 'M'

For more on myocardial infarction, see p. 212

Q waves and inverted T waves (ECG 5)

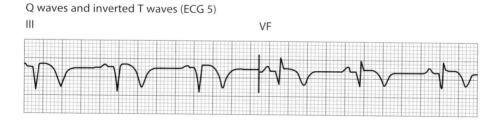

'M' pattern (ECG 6)

V₆

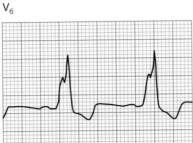

ECG 7

The ECG shows:

- Atrial fibrillation
- Normal axis
- Normal QRS complexes
- Downward-sloping ST segments, best seen in leads V_4–V_6
- U waves, best seen in lead V_2

Interpretation of the ECG

The completely irregular rhythm with narrow QRS complexes must be due to atrial fibrillation, even though the usual baseline irregularity is not very obvious. The downward-sloping ST segments indicate that she is taking digoxin, which explains the good control of the ventricular rate (with untreated atrial fibrillation the ventricular rate would usually be rapid), and the U waves suggest hypokalaemia (see the extracts from the traces, opposite page: in lead V_5 the downward-sloping ST segment is arrowed).

If you made a mistake with this one, read p. 101.

ECG
IP

For more on the ECG in patients with dizziness, see Ch. 2

pattern, best seen in the lateral leads (see the extract from lead V_6, above) shows that this is left bundle branch block (LBBB). In LBBB the T waves are usually inverted in the lateral leads, and have no further significance. In the presence of LBBB the ECG cannot be interpreted any further, so it is not possible to comment on the presence or absence of ischaemia.

If you need to check, look at pp. 43 and 45.

Clinical management

The story sounds like angina, but when angina is combined with dizziness always think of aortic stenosis, which can also cause angina even with normal coronary arteries. LBBB is common in aortic stenosis. A patient with aortic stenosis who is dizzy on exertion has a high risk of sudden death, and this patient needs urgent investigation with a view to early aortic valve replacement.

ECG
IP

For more on electrolyte abnormalities, see p. 331

Clinical management

If this patient who is taking digoxin feels sick she is probably suffering from digoxin toxicity and hypokalaemia may be the main cause of this. Hypokalaemia is likely to occur if a patient with heart failure is given a loop diuretic without either a potassium-retaining diuretic or potassium supplements. The serum potassium

U wave and downward-sloping ST segment (ECG 7)

V₂

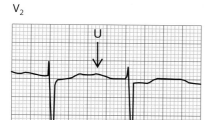

V₅

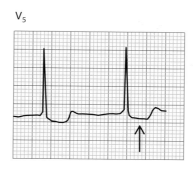

For more on normal variants of the ECG, see Ch. 1

For more on diagnosis of left ventricular hypertrophy, see pp. 295–303

level must be checked urgently, and appropriate action taken.

Remember that we have still not made a full diagnosis: what is the cause of the atrial fibrillation? Most cardiac conditions can be associated with atrial fibrillation, but in elderly patients the important disease to remember is thyrotoxicosis, because atrial fibrillation may be the only manifestation of this in the elderly.

ECG 8

This ECG shows:

- Sinus rhythm
- Bifid P waves
- Normal conducting intervals

- Normal axis
- Tall R wave in lead V₅ and deep S wave in lead V₂
- Small (septal) Q wave in leads I, VL and V₅–V₆
- Inverted T waves in leads I, VL and V₅–V₆
- U waves in leads V₂–V₄ (normal).

Interpretation of the ECG

The bifid P waves, best seen in lead V₃, indicate left atrial hypertrophy (see the extracts from the trace, p. 192). The combined height of the R wave in lead V₅ plus the depth of the S wave in lead V₂ is 58 mm, so there are 'voltage criteria' for left ventricular hypertrophy. The inverted T waves in the lateral leads confirm severe left ventricular hypertrophy. The Q waves

191

P wave and R wave (ECG 8)

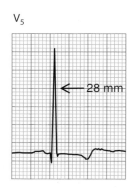

V_3 V_5

P

← 28 mm

are small and narrow, and are therefore septal in origin and do not indicate an old infarction.

If you needed help with this one, re-read pp. 90–91.

Clinical management

This patient has clinical and ECG evidence of left ventricular hypertrophy, but this is not a full diagnosis – what might be the cause of the hypertension? A young man with hypertension who has abnormal pulses in the legs almost certainly has a coarctation of the aorta, which needs investigation and correction.

ECG 9

This ECG shows:

- Narrow QRS complexes (duration less than 120 ms)
- Tachycardia at 200/min

- No visible P waves
- Normal QRS complexes
- ST segments with a little depression in leads II, III and VF
- Normal T waves except in lead III.

Interpretation of the ECG

The QRS complexes are narrow, so this is a supraventricular tachycardia. It is regular, so it is not atrial fibrillation. No P waves are visible so it is not sinus rhythm, atrial tachycardia or atrial flutter (see the extract from the trace below). This has to be an AV nodal re-entry or junctional, tachycardia (sometimes, but not logically, referred to as 'supraventricular tachycardia or 'SVT').

In case of difficulty, look at pp. 70–71.

Narrow QRS complexes and no visible P waves (ECG 9)

V_3

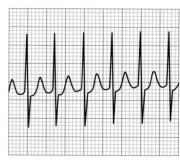

Clinical management

This rhythm can often be terminated by carotid sinus pressure, or by the Valsalva manoeuvre. Failing that, it will usually respond to intravenous adenosine. DC cardioversion should be considered for any patient with tachycardia that is compromising the circulation. The best way of preventing the attacks depends on their frequency and severity. An electrophysiological study, with a view to possible ablation of an abnormal conducting pathway, should be considered.

ECG 10

This ECG shows:

- Sinus rhythm
- Normal conducting intervals
- Normal axis
- Small R waves in leads V_1–V_2
- Very small R wave in lead V_3
- Small Q wave and very small R wave in lead V_4
- Raised ST segments in leads I, VL and V_2–V_5.

Interpretation of the ECG

The small R waves in leads V_1–V_2 could be normal, but leads V_3–V_4 should show larger R waves. The raised ST segments indicate an ST segment elevation myocardial infarction (see the extracts from the traces, oposite). The small Q wave in lead V_4 suggests that a fairly short time has elapsed since the onset of the infarction, and

this Q wave will probably become larger over the next few hours. Since the changes are limited to leads I, VL and V_2–V_5, this is an acute anterolateral myocardial infarction (STEMI).

You must have got this one right – the ECG is easy!

Clinical management

This man needs urgent pain relief. Pain radiating to the back always raises the possibility of an aortic dissection, but it is quite common in acute infarction, and there are no physical signs – loss of pulses, asymmetric blood pressure in the arms, a murmur of aortic regurgitation or pericarditis – to support a diagnosis of aortic dissection. If in doubt an urgent echocardiogram may help, but essentially this patient needs either immediate thrombolysis or angioplasty.

The moral of this story – and of all the others – is that an ECG is an aid to diagnosis, not a substitute for further thought.

For more on electrophysiology and ablation, see pp. 155–162

For more on myocardial infarction, see pp. 214–246

R wave and Q wave (ECG 10)

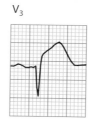

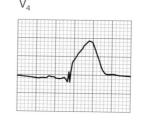

V_3 V_4

If you find testing yourself helpful, try 150 ECG Problems

193

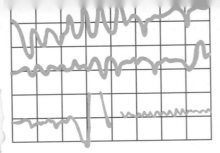

Index

Note: Page numbers in **bold** refer to figures and tables.
Abbreviations used in subentries: LBBB, left bundle branch block; RBBB, right bundle branch block.

Index

Index